A POCKETBOOK OF SOCIAL AND COMMUNITY PAEDIATRICS

KV-191-217

Jo Sibert MD, FRCP, DCH

*Professor of Community Child Health,
University of Wales College of Medicine, Cardiff.*

Edward Arnold
A division of Hodder & Stoughton
LONDON   MELBOURNE   AUCKLAND

© 1992 J.R. Sibert

First published in Great Britain 1992

British Library Cataloguing-in-Publication Data
Sibert, Jo
    A pocket book of social and community paediatrics
    I. Title
    362.7

ISBN 0-340-54929-7

Typeset in 10/11 Times by Hewer Text Composition Services, Edinburgh.
Printed and bound in Great Britain for Edward Arnold, the
educational, academic and medical division of Hodder and
Stoughton Limited, Mill Road, Dunton Green, Sevenoaks,
Kent TN13 2YA by Clays Ltd, St Ives plc, Bungay, Suffolk.

This book is dedicated to my wife Sue and to my children Ben, Dan, Tom, Rebecca and Matthew from whom I have learnt much about child health and development.

Contents

Preface

When I was a junior doctor I was very much helped by guides
to clinical practice that could be carried around with me.
These guides gave much detail on the problems of treating
the acutely ill child but were of much less help on the wider
issues of the social background of the family and how the
child should be cared for in the community. This book tries
to fill that gap. I hope it will provide a practical, easy-to-carry
guide for doctors and other health care professionals working
with children both in the community and in the hospital. I
also hope it will be of value to medical students.

The book provides guidance on how to take a history and
conduct an examination so as to be in a position to help the
child and family best, and it provides information on benefits
and housing that may be available for them. The difficult
subject of child abuse and how it should be dealt with is
covered in what I hope is a practical way. Many doctors
find all the legal aspects of caring for children daunting; in
particular giving evidence in court. I hope this book will help
them. The *Children Act* 1989 will make important differences
to child care and is covered not only in its impact on child
abuse but also divorce.

Sudden infant death syndrome is the commonest cause of
death in children between the age of a month and a year,
and accidents in children the commonest cause of death in
children over the age of a year. The prevention of both these
problems is now seen as a priority in community child health

and is covered in this book. Children spend much of their time at school and this book aims to help doctors relate to the problems they face in school. Our role in immunization programmes is also covered.

The child surveillance programme has changed the way we detect problems and talk to parents in the first five years of a child's life. This book covers all aspects of the programme and how we deal with problems. This includes behavioural problems, children with special needs and non-organic problems.

I hope particularly that the approach of this book will be suitable for work in the hospital and community and in a small way will help the creation of the integrated child health service that many of us wish will be created soon throughout the country.

J.R. Sibert MA, MD, B.Chir,
FRCP, DCH, D.Obst RCOG
1991

Acknowledgements

I would like to thank my colleagues for their advice and support during the preparation of this book, in particular, Dr Paul Davis, Dr Annette Davies, Dr Rosemary Isaac, Dr Elspeth Webb and Mrs Val Winter.

1 Introduction

Taking a social paediatric history

All doctors caring for children, whether in hospital or in the community, need to be able to take a history which is going to be useful in coming to a diagnosis and assessing the needs of the child and family. This should be in two main parts:

1. The basic data about the child and the family
2. The problems that are presenting at that time

Basic data on a child

The basic data on a child should include:

- Birth data – where, were there any problems, birthweight?
- Past history – any hospital admissions, which immunizations have been given?
- Family data – the age of parents, their occupation, state of health, were there any diseases in family?
- A family tree is useful in many cases particularly if there are complex family relationships or genetic diseases.
- If there is divorce or separation does the child see both parents?
- Development – have simple milestones been achieved?

● School – where, have there been any changes of school, is school work adequate, has school work changed?

Problem lists

Problem lists provide an essential tool in the assessment and management of children with social and community problems.

When the concept of problem-orientated medical records was first suggested each entry should have been under the headings subjective, objective, analysis, plans (SOAP). Such a detailed analysis may not be necessary in most cases, however, it is important to recognize individual problems and to formulate plans.

A problem list presents an ideal heading to any correspondence about the child and provides an ideal basis for any future consultations.

Making a problem list

Usually the presenting problem is considered first. It is important also to mention parental concern, whether justified or not, and concerns such as about developmental problems, social problems and housing.

A typical list might be:

1. Neurofibromatosis
2. Social concern and concern regarding neglect
3. Speech delay
4. Housing problem
5. Parental concern regarding short stature

Talking to parents

Talking to parents is a skill which is acquired with difficulty by all those looking after children. Many parents are unhappy in medical situations, whether it is in a hospital, in a community clinic or in the GP's surgery, and need putting at ease. If they are at ease then the child will be at ease too. It is therefore important to discuss the family situation in a calm and relaxed manner before going on to particular problems.

It is very difficult to expect parents fully to comprehend and discuss major and difficult diagnoses such as Duchenne muscular dystrophy and Down's syndrome on the first hearing. It is also difficult for them to be told such information and expect them to go home on the bus. Home visits enable parents to be put at ease and be able to discuss the prognosis and treatment with relatives.

Examination

All children seen initially need to be examined. What needs to be examined depends very much on the circumstances. Many toddlers hate to be examined. Much can be learnt on development from observing the children. A child-friendly environment is essential for this with toys and pictures for them to see. Small children are best examined on the lap.

Is the child thriving and is the child developing?

• All children seen by doctors should have their growth assessed. This will mean accurate weighing, which means not only accurate scales but a standard degree of undressing. Babies under a year old need to be naked if the weight is to have any value.
• Length needs to be measured in babies in a neonatometer or some other accurate method of measuring. A tape measure is not sufficient and very inaccurate. Older children need a height gauge.
• Head circumference should be measured in all children under two years of age and in certain children over two.
• Development should be assessed in all children seen.

What help is needed and what help is the family getting?

At the end of a consultation with a doctor an assessment should be made on the needs of the child. These needs and plans should be made relevant to individual problems.

Most children suffering from child abuse, with development and behaviour problems and children with special needs have many professionals involved in their cases. This can be very confusing for parents. It is important to have clear medical leadership. The GP has a major role in complicated cases as does the consultant paediatrician (community child health).

Prevention

Every child who is seen for medical assessment, particularly in the community setting, should have a clear assessment of what scope there is for prevention of disease.

This should include:

- Infectious disease, in particular making a note of immunizations
- Genetic disease
- Accidents
- Asthma
- Tooth decay
- Dietary considerations

2 Helping the child and the family

Health care professionals

Which particular health care professional a child may see for a particular problem varies from area to area, however, there are general principles that do apply, such as working together in a team. It is sometimes quite difficult to decide the best mode of referral for children. Those who may be involved include:

Doctors

General practitioners

Clearly GPs have the lead role in the primary care of children and have an increasing role in child surveillance.

Paediatricians

Paediatricians may be based in the hospital, in the community or both. They have a particular role in coordinating a multidisciplinary team. They are involved in the assessment of child and family, and investigations and treatment of problems raised by child surveillance. They may provide a service in cases of child abuse.

Paediatric neurologists

The investigation and diagnosis of specific neurological problems in childhood are dealt with by paediatric neurologists.

Community paediatric staff

Senior clinical medical officers and clinical medical officers have a varied role in Child Health Services, particularly in the School Medical Service, Audiology Services and special developmental assessment.

Paediatric surgeons

Paediatric surgeons deal with surgical conditions in childhood which include hernias, undescended testes, etc. Most paediatric surgeons deal with urological problems in childhood although in some districts these are dealt with by urologists. They also deal with hypospadias although sometimes plastic surgeons deal with this problem.

Ear, nose and throat surgeons

Specialist help is given by ear, nose and throat surgeons for cases of hearing and ear problems together with tonsillectomy.

Orthopaedic surgeons

Specialist assessment of congenital dislocation of the hip, talipes and scoliosis is done by orthopaedic surgeons. Minor orthopaedic problems can often be dealt with by the consultant paediatrician in community child health or the GP.

Plastic surgeons

Cosmetic problems such as polydactyly and accessory auricles are dealt with by plastic surgeons. They also deal with burns and scalds, cleft lip and palate and in some centres hypospadias.

Specialists in accident and emergency medicine

Specialists in accident and emergency medicine deal with children in the Accident and Emergency Department. Some centres now have specialists in paediatric accident and emergency medicine.

Medical geneticists

A specialist genetic counselling service is provided by medical geneticists for families and in most centres a dysmorphology service.

Child psychiatrists

Emotional problems and psychiatric disease in childhood such as anorexia nervosa are dealt with by child psychiatrists. They particularly deal with the assessment of emotional abuse.

Dentists

General dental practitioners

The general dental practitioners deal with the majority of dental problems in childhood.

Community dentists

Community dentists treat some children in school and they review general dental policy.

Specialists in paediatric dentistry

They provide a specialist service based in the hospital and community.

Orthodontic surgeons

Cosmetic problems in relation to teeth are dealt with by orthodontic surgeons. They provide a specialist role in cleft lip and palate cases.

Therapists

Therapists dealing with children with special needs should be part of a multidisciplinary team. The differences between the individual disciplines in therapy are becoming blurred.

Physiotherapists

Physiotherapists have a role in the physical treatment of disease, in particular with cerebral palsy and in newborns. They also deal with other physical handicaps such as muscular dystrophy.

Occupational therapists

Therapy directed to what children do is given by occupational therapists. They have a particular role in dealing with clumsy children, home adaptions and assessment for disabled living and for the assessment of children for wheelchairs.

Speech therapists

Speech therapists give a specialist assessment of speech and language problems. They also deal with problems in swallowing.

Other therapists

The role of play therapists and music therapists is not yet established. Their training is not at present recognized by the National Health Service.

Nurses

Health visitors

Health visitors are now attached to the primary care team and have special responsibilities for children. They undertake a major part of the child surveillance programme.

Paediatric trained nurses (registered sick children nurses, RSCN)

These nurses have a role mainly in hospital but increasingly in the community.

Nursery nurses (nursery nurse examination board, NNEB)

These nurses have an important role in caring and playing with children in hospitals, nurseries, playgroups and schools.

Other health care professionals

Dietitians

Dietitians deal with dietary problems in children. Their assessment of iron intake in anaemia is valuable in the community setting.

Audiological scientists

These scientists deal with the accurate assessment of hearing in children.

Child psychologists

Behavioural problems in childhood are dealt with by child psychologists. The interface with child psychiatry is different in different areas. Many are involved with developmental problems in children, particularly in supervising the Home Advisory Service or Portage System.

Home advisors

Home advisors are involved in the day-to-day running of the Home Advisory Service.

Orthotists

Orthotists fit and supply orthoses which are appliances fitted externally to support or correct a deformity.

Bioengineers

Bioengineers may be involved in specific areas of seating and wheelchairs in childhood.

Teachers and other professionals in school

Teachers in primary and secondary schools

These teachers are an important source of information on children.

Educational psychologists

Educational psychologists assess children's abilities and progress at school. They are involved very much in preparing statements for children with special needs. Sometimes they are involved with behavioural problems in childhood as they present to school.

Specialist advisory teachers

These teachers advise on groups of children such as the visually and hearing impaired. They are often involved from the pre-school period.

Social workers

The Social Services Department has a director, who is responsible to the Social Services Committee of the County Council or London or Metropolitan Borough. He or she works with a number of assistant directors. Usually one of the assistant directors is concerned with children and families and has a particular relevance for doctors working with children. Social workers are usually divided into teams often locally based, with a principal social services officer in charge of each district.

Social workers dealing with children are employed by the Local Authority and may be involved with:

- Work with children and families, in particular child protection
- Work in the hospital
- Work with the physically handicapped
- Work with adoption and fostering
- Work with the mentally ill

Social workers may also work for other agencies:

- The National Society for the Prevention of Cruelty to Children (NSPCC) has a statutory role in protecting children. In individual areas they may also have a heavy case load or may undertake more specialized functions (e.g. maintaining the Child Protection Register).

• The National Children's Home (NCH) has an increasing role in child abuse cases, but does not have a statutory role. They are involved with local nurseries and projects preventing child abuse in several parts of the country.

• Barnardo's is now involved in local projects with deprived children. It is also involved with Link Families for Children with Special Needs.

• Save the Children is involved in running nurseries for deprived children in certain areas.

Housing

Indifferent housing presents a major problem for many children and their families. Doctors working with children are often asked for help in housing families. Social workers and the Citizens' Advice Bureau will usually be able to advise on this.

Council housing

This is dealt with by District Councils London and Metropolitan Boroughs and their Housing Departments. The person usually responsible is the director of housing. Waiting lists are dealt with on a points system with points being awarded for the number of children, state of the present property, etc. There are usually points awarded for medical need.

Housing associations

Housing associations may provide housing in some areas. Often they have links with the local Council waiting list. There may be specialist housing association property for the disabled.

Private rented accommodation

This is usually found by searching locally. The social worker or Citizens' Advice Bureau can help.

goes to work. It does not depend on the national insurance record.

The amount of family credit depends on the family's income.

Family credit can be claimed using a form FC1 Family Credit available from main Post Offices.

If the family is eligible for family credit they may be able to get help with NHS costs. There is a special maternity payment from the Social Fund, a funeral payment from the Social Fund and also help with rent and Community Charge.

Income support

Income support is a benefit to help people who do not have enough money to live on. To receive income support the claimant must be aged over 18 years and has to be working less than 24 hours a week. They must not have more than £6000 in savings.

Income support is made up of a personal allowance, premiums for groups of people with special needs and housing costs payments.

The income support claim forms are found at Unemployment Benefit Offices.

Housing benefit

Housing benefit is paid by local councils to people on low incomes who are paying rent and Community Charge.

Housing benefit is not paid to help with mortgage interest payments, fuel costs or meals.

Families on low income who pay rent and Community Charge may be able to receive housing benefit.

The benefit is calculated according to earnings, unearned income and savings.

Claim forms are obtainable through the local councils.

Help with National Health Service costs

If a family is on family credit or income support they automatically qualify for free NHS prescriptions, free NHS sight tests, refund of travel costs to hospital for NHS treatment and free NHS wigs and fabric supports.

If a family is on low income but not eligible for family credit they may be eligible for a refund of NHS costs. A form AG1 can be obtained from the Social Security Office for this.

Social Fund

The Social Fund helps people with exceptional expenses which are difficult to pay for out of regular income. These benefits include maternity benefit, funeral payment, cold weather payments, community care grants, budgeting loans and crisis loans.

Forms for these benefits are available through Social Security Offices.

One parent benefit

One parent benefit is available to families with a single, divorced, widowed or separated parent bringing up a child on their own. The weekly benefit is paid for one child only, usually the first.

The same rate applies on no matter what you earn or how large the family. The claim form is CH11 One Parent Benefit.

Widow's benefit

When a father dies the widow may be able to receive a widow's payment and also a widowed mother's allowance.

Statutory maternity pay

Pregnant women may be able to claim a weekly payment from their employer. If a pregnant woman is not able to claim statutory maternity pay, maternity allowance would be payable from the Department of Social Security or maybe from Social Fund maternity payments.

Unemployment benefit

This benefit is available for those who are capable of and available for work on every day for which the claim is made.

The unemployed should contact the local Unemployment Benefit Office on the first day that unemployment starts. Their P45 tax form will be needed for claiming.

Guardian's allowance

If a person is looking after an orphaned child as part of a family a guardian's allowance may be payable. Both of the child's parents may be dead, or one dead and the other one missing, in prison or divorced. They do not have to be the legal guardian, but do have to be entitled to child benefit for the child.

The child in care

If a child goes into care child benefit will stop after 8 weeks unless he or she goes home regularly.

Benefits available to families with children with special needs

Attendance Allowance and Mobility Allowance

These benefits are replaced from April 1992 by Disability Living Allowance.

Disability Living Allowance

Disability Living Allowance is a tax free benefit for care of mobility need from a disability or illness. It has two components:

The Care Component which replaces the Attendance Allowance. It has no lower age limit and is payable from the age of three months. It may be at three rates:

- Higher Rate for 24 hour attention or supervision.
- Mid Rate for attention or supervision either day or night.
- Lower Rate for those people who need attention or supervision for part of the day.

Mobility Component which replaces mobility allowance and is payable from the age of five years. It may be at two rates.

- Higher Rate for those who do not walk or are virtually unable to walk.
- Lower Rate for those who are able to walk but need guidance or supervision.

The Disability Living Allowance unlike Attendance and Mobility Allowances will be assessed initially on a statement from the family on a claim pack. Special medical examination will not normally be necessary.

Invalid care allowance

Parents who spend much of their time looking after a disabled child who receives an attendance allowance may be eligible for invalid care allowance. The carer must spend 35 hours every week from Sunday to Saturday caring for the disabled patient. If the carer stops looking after the disabled patient for a short time they are still eligible for the allowance, for example, when a short holiday is taken or when the patient goes into hospital. There can be a total of 12 weeks break in any 6-month period.

Severe disablement allowance

If a child is sick or disabled, aged 16 years or over and is incapable of work, the severe disablement allowance may be payable.

Joseph Rowntree Memorial Trust

The Joseph Rowntree Memorial Trust administers the Family Fund. This is based in York and gives grants to severely disabled children and their families. Their address is:

Joseph Rowntree Memorial Trust
PO Box 50
York YO1 2ZX
UK

Paediatricians in hospitals and in the community are often asked for reports on children for this fund.

The social worker would be able to advise on claiming from this fund which is funded by the government.

Helping children from ethnic minorities

The recognition of the social structure of ethnic minority groups is important in helping children and their families. There is often misunderstanding by doctors about different ethnic minority groups, particularly those from the Indian sub-continent, regarding religion, diet and any particular health problems. Literature for parents should be produced in relevant ethnic minority languages.

A broad outline of the main ethnic minority groups in the UK and the particular health problems that they may suffer from are discussed in Table 2.1.

Table 2.1 Potential health problems which may be experienced by members of different ethnic groups.

Ethnic groups	Area of ethnic origin	Potential health problems
Afro-Caribbean	West Indies (most in the UK are second or third generation Britons)	Rastafarian children may be vegetarian. Sickle cell anaemia
Indian Gujerati (religion=Hindu; language=Gujerati)	Indian state of Gujerat or Bombay, East Africa, Kenya, Uganda	Diet may be low in vitamin D and lead to rickets with inadequate exposure to sunlight Thalassaemia
Sikhs (religion=Sikhism)	Indian state of Punjab	Rickets

Ethnic groups	Area of ethnic origin	Potential health problems
Punjabi Muslims (language=Urdu or Punjabi)	Pakistani region of Punjab	Thalassaemia and rickets. Consanguinuity is common with an increased risk of congenital malformation
Pathans (religion=Muslim; language=Pashtu)	North west frontier province of Pakistan	Thalassaemia
Bengalis (religion=Muslim; language=Bengali)	Bangladesh	Many families live in poverty
Tamils (religion=Hindu, Christian; language =Tamil)	South India Sri Lanka	Consanguinity Thalassaemia
African Somalis	Somalia	Sickle cell anaemia. Female circumcision?
Nigerian (religion=Christian or Muslim)	Nigeria	Sickle cell anaemia
Yemeni Muslims	Yemen	Iron deficiency, anaemia and rickets
Jews Ashkenazi	Eastern Europe	Rare recessively inherited diseases, e.g. Tay-Sachs disease, Riley Day syndrome and Gauchers disease
Sephardic	Middle East	Not a numerous group in Britain
Chinese (language=Cantonese)	Hong Kong	Glucose-6-phosphate dehydrogenase deficiency

3 Dealing with child abuse

Many doctors find dealing with children who may have been abused difficult and indeed some cases present many problems. The keys to success in this field are

- Take a history and examination like any other patient so that the whole consultation is put firmly within a medical framework. This has a calming effect on the parents and child.
- Work in a multidisciplinary way getting mutual support from everyone involved in the case including social workers, the police, health visitors etc.
- Always record the findings of the case in detail in the notes. Injuries should be measured.
- If in doubt get a second opinion.

Sometimes child abuse is thought of as 'the battered baby'. Although some babies are injured very severely, abuse can occur at any age during childhood and to both boys and girls. Child abuse can also occur both in rich and poor families. We do know, however, that there are certain factors that do predispose to child abuse. These include:

- Young mothers
- Low social class and unemployment
- Marital instability
- Pre-term babies
- Low birth weight

- Indifferent housing
- Alcohol

We also know that if a child has been abused once he or she is much more likely to be abused again than other children. Recognizing this is very important in the prevention of abuse. Serious injuries to children only rarely come as the first episode and are almost always preceded by more minor injuries.

Patterns of child abuse

Although children do present with a single type of abuse, it is more common for children to suffer from a pattern of abuse, i.e. physically abused children are often neglected and emotionally abused. Abuse of all types is very damaging to the emotional development of the child. Sexual abuse may also damage the future sexual responses of a girl or boy. We should aim not only to prevent further injuries but to prevent further emotional damage to a child. All abused children need a full medical assessment, a developmental assessment and a behavioural assessment.

Types of abuse

- Physical abuse (which may include bruises, burns, lacerations, fractures and internal injuries)
- Neglect (which may include non-organic failure to thrive, developmental delay, non-attendance at school etc.)
- Emotional abuse (which may present as behavioural problems, scapegoating etc.)
- Sexual abuse
- Non-accidental poisoning (where children are deliberately poisoned)
- The Munchausen syndrome by proxy (where symptoms or signs are fabricated)

Dealing with a patient with suspected child abuse

Abused children may present in a variety of different ways.

They may present in ordinary clinical practice such as in the Accident and Emergency Department, General Practice or the community. They may also be brought for a medical opinion by the social services department or the police.

In all cases the procedures of the local Area Child Protection Committee should be followed. These may be rather different in sexual abuse cases than in physical abuse cases.

If a possibly abused child is examined under that procedure the consultation should take place just as if the child had an ordinary medical condition – with a full history being taken and an examination. The consultation should take place in a child-friendly place such as a children's centre if at all possible. Any injuries should be carefully noted, measured, recorded and drawn on a topographical chart. The height and weight should be recorded and put on a percentile chart. An attempt should be made to assess the development.

If there are significant injuries photographs should be taken for medico-legal purposes by a photographer who is willing to give evidence in court if necessary. Sometimes photographs of bruises do not do justice to the severity of the injuries.

If, after the examination, abuse is confirmed or if there is a need for further investigation a decision needs to be made whether the child needs protection as an emergency measure. This should be done in consultation with the social workers involved in the case who may consult the senior social worker on duty.

Protection of the child is usually achieved by admission to hospital, which also allows investigations, but may be by admission to a children's home or foster home. If at all possible such admissions should be on a voluntary basis but sometimes legal action is needed (see the section on the law, p. 36).

Dealing with a patient with suspected child sexual abuse

Procedures may be rather different in sexual abuse cases than in physical abuse cases where a preliminary investigation with the involvement of the police and social services should take place before the medical examination.

Full details are discussed in the chapter on sexual abuse.

The Case Conference

If child abuse is confirmed or suspected a Case Conference will be held under the local Area Child Protection Committee procedure. This will be under the guidelines laid down by the Department of Health. The Conference will be chaired by a senior member of the Social Services Department or NSPCC. Members of the Conference will include social workers, health visitors and nurses, the police, the GP, paediatricians, teachers and lawyers. Guidance under the Children Act 1989 (Working Together) clearly implies that parents and older children should be allowed to attend case conferences. They should now only be excluded at the decision of the Chairman.

If you examined a child who may have been abused **do go to the Case Conference**. It may be the only opportunity you have of putting your views forward and protecting the child. You may also be able to claim a fee from the Health Authority.

The General Medical Council regards it as the duty of doctors to disclose confidential information if it is in the interest of the child in such circumstances.

At the Conference details of the incident leading to the Conference and the family background will be discussed. The Conference will decide whether to place the child's name on the Child Protection Register, whether there should be an application to the Juvenile Court to protect the child and what follow-up is needed. The Social Services Department will have to develop a Child Protection Plan which should include medical follow-up in many cases.

When talking to the Conference give the details of the examination and your involvement with the child. A written report is most helpful. Give your opinion on the case and give your views on whether the child should be protected, what further tests are needed and what medical follow-up is needed.

If you disagree very much with the conclusions of the Case Conference, write, stating your views, to the Director of Social Services in the area in which the child lives with a copy to the Chair of the Conference.

Medical follow-up

Medical follow-up is increasingly being recognized as part of the management of child abuse. This is to:

- Monitor growth
- Monitor behaviour
- Monitor development – in particular speech delay
- Record further injuries

This information is important when giving evidence in court and important in helping the Social Services Department to come to a conclusion on management.

The Social Services will have to prepare a Child Protection Plan. Medical follow-up should be part of that plan in most cases. It should also be part of any contract with the parents of the child.

Further Reading

Working Together under the Children Act, 1989. HMSO, London.

4 Recognition of child abuse

The recognition of child abuse is essentially a sum of probabilities that individual injuries or harm that the child has suffered has occurred non-accidentally. Late presentation and a story which does not fit the facts are all suggestive of abuse.

Physical abuse

Bruises

Bruises are the commonest presentation of physical abuse. Sometimes a clear hand, shoe or stick mark can be seen. Generally one needs to be confident however that the combination of injuries one observes could not have been the result of a single accident. Bruises should be always considered as a whole and not singly.

There are some areas of the body that if bruised are particularly suggestive of abuse. Bruises on the face (which is protected by the nose and eyebrow from accidental injury), the back, abdomen and the buttocks are all suggestive of abuse. Multiple bruises on the upper arm and upper thighs are also suggestive of abuse.

Bruises on the shins are common in all children and should usually be ignored. Bruises on the forehead are also commonly caused accidentally.

Bruises on the genitalia, the upper thigh or lower abdomen should alert one to the possibility of sexual abuse.

Coagulation disorders should be excluded in cases due to bruising for medico-legal reasons. A coagulation screen performed by the haematological laboratory is the best way of doing this. This will include: platelets, prothrombin time and kaolin cephalin clotting time.

Fractures

Fractures caused non-accidentally in children under the age of 3 years may be difficult to detect clinically. They should be excluded in potentially abused children under 3 years by skeletal survey X-rays and isotope bone scan. Skeletal survey will detect old fractures and isotope bone scan will detect some recent fractures that do not show up on X-rays. Fractures in children over 3 years will present clinically and do not generally need X-rays.

All fractures can be caused in a non-accidental way but some fractures are more likely to be caused non-accidentally than others. These include:

- Fractured ribs (which are caused by squeezing rather than direct trauma and are usually posterior).
- Spiral fractures of long bones in children under two years. Spiral fractures of the humerus in babies are almost always due to abuse. These are caused by twisting.
- Metaphyseal fractures of long bones caused by wrenching.

Excluding osteogenesis imperfecta

Sometimes osteogenesis imperfecta may present as child abuse (see p. 000). Although there is no doubt this does rarely occur, the possibility is often brought up by lawyers representing the family in such cases. This diagnosis therefore needs exclusion in fractures in children thought to be due to abuse.

Osteogenesis imperfecta type I

This is dominantly inherited and a full family history should be taken. There are blue sclerae on examination. Skeletal survey may show reduced bone density and multiple wormian bones on the skull film. Normal children often have several wormian bones on skull X-ray. The wormian bones on skull X-ray in osteogenesis imperfecta are multiple and occupy the whole bone structure in a mosaic pattern.

Osteogenesis imperfecta types II and III

Type II is lethal and Type III gives severe deformity.

Osteogenesis imperfecta type IV

This presents with white sclerae and is dominantly inherited. Type IV has been suggested as a common differential diagnosis in child abuse, however, it is:

- Very rare
- Associated with deformity
- Associated with reduced bone density

Copper deficiency

Copper deficiency has also been suggested as a differential diagnosis of child abuse. This is very unlikely as there is adequate copper in breast milk and in all the formula feeds available in the UK. The only group of children who might be deficient in copper are pre-term babies who have been parentally fed. Copper deficiency presents as much more than increased bone fragility. There will also be developmental delay, sparse hair, anaemia and dry skin as well.

Despite copper deficiency being extremely rare and being able to be recognized on clinical grounds, the possibility is sometimes brought up by lawyers representing the family in abuse cases. It is therefore wise to check the serum and urinary copper and serum caeruloplasmin in such cases.

Bites

Adult bite marks may be seen in abused children. The important differential diagnosis is from a child's bite or animal bites. The forensic dentist may be useful in the assessment of these injuries. He or she may be able to take imprints from potential abusers' mouths to help with the exact diagnosis. Photographs should be taken at an early stage.

Burns

Burns and scalds can be caused non-accidentally. The diagnosis may be difficult in such cases.

The history is particularly important and details of exactly how the burn or scald was said to have been caused should be carefully recorded. There should be an assessment of whether this explanation could explain the injury. The forensic department of the police may be helpful in calculating the physics of a possible cause of a burn.

The site of the burn is important: scalds on the back are difficult to cause in an accidental way. Sometimes a mark such as a tip of an iron or the bars of a fire can be seen.

Many children present with possible cigarette burns. These are punched out lesions the diameter of a cigarette. They cannot be caused by brushing against the skin with a lighted cigarette. They need pressure on the skin to be caused. A common differential diagnosis is staphylococcal bullous impetigo, where the lesions are of different sizes.

Neglect and emotional abuse

The recognition of neglect and emotional abuse is important. Although some children are permanently damaged by physical abuse, the numbers are relatively small. However, very many children have their personalities damaged after neglect and emotional abuse. The assessment of neglect is not a purely medical one. Often evidence of the state of the home, that the child is always hungry and that he or she is never properly clothed is more important than the medical evidence.

Neglect may present medically as:

● *Failure to thrive* with weight gain across percentile lines in hospital or in care. Every possibly abused child should be put on a percentile chart. Extensive investigation is not necessary although simple tests, i.e. full blood count, urine and stool culture should be checked.

● *Speech and developmental delay.* Many abused children have delayed milestones. The development should be assessed informally in all abuse cases. If there is any doubt about the milestones a Griffith's test should be performed. There is sometimes a need for a speech therapist's assessment.

● *Poor standard of care and cleanliness.* The state of the child when assessed should always be noted. Significant physical signs include:

(a) Severe nappy rash which will have punched out ulcers from chronically infrequent nappy changes.

(b) 'Urine burn' – acute erythema of the napkin area and legs from acute non-changing of nappies.

(c) Dirty finger nails in babies.

(d) Red extremities. Red hands and feet are often found in neglected children under the age of 5 years. This resolves very quickly when they are taken into a satisfactory environment. It is probably due to autonomic disturbance.

● *Poor attendance at school.* Neglected children often are not presented for school and have a poor attendance record. A school report is often valuable.

● *Accidents.* Neglected children may present with frequent preventable accidents.

● *Poor attendance for medical attention.* Neglected children are often not presented for medical appointments, immunizations etc. A clear record of this is valuable in the assessment of children.

All these features improve with nothing else but changing the child's environment in neglect.

Emotional abuse

Many physically abused children and neglected children are emotionally abused as well. Children need love and understanding to develop normally. In emotional abuse there may be:

- The withdrawal of love for the child and rejection
- Criticism, threat and ridicule
- Unusual, unreasonable and cruel punishment
- Scapegoating where one child is much favoured over another

Emotional abuse may present as:

- Behaviour disturbances such as temper tantrums
- A withdrawn sad child
- Depression
- Poor school work and underperformance

If emotional abuse is suspected there should be an assessment by a child psychiatrist or psychologist.

Non-accidental poisoning

Some children are deliberately poisoned by their parents or others. They present with bizarre symptoms rather than poisoning directly. Accidental child poisoning is a common problem in toddlers and is related to stress but by definition is accidental.

The diagnosis in non-accidental poisoning is made by finding the drug concerned in the blood or urine.

Children may present with such symptoms as:

- Hyperventilation after salicylates
- Unexplained sedation after hypnotics, tranquillizers or alcohol
- Thirst after poisoning with common salt

Munchausen syndrome by proxy

In this syndrome symptoms and signs are deliberately fabricated to bring the child under medical attention by a parent (usually the mother who is psychologically disturbed). This can be very damaging to the child not only because there is often unnecessary investigation but also because dangerous treatment can be given. The child also has to live with a pattern of illness rather than health.

Symptoms and signs that can be fabricated may include:

- Blood in the vomit, stool and urine
- Placing glucose in the urine so that a diagnosis of diabetes is made
- Deliberately infecting microbiological specimens
- Fits

5 Sexual abuse

Dealing with a patient with suspected child sexual abuse

Procedures may be rather different in sexual abuse cases than in physical abuse cases and where a preliminary investigation with the involvement of the police and social services should take place before the medical examination. If in doubt consult your local Procedure Book of the Area Child Protection Committee.

There is rarely any hurry in child sexual abuse cases. It is much better to pause and plan rather than rush into medical examination. Attempts at disclosure work are best not done by doctors unless they have considerable time to follow the situation.

Who should be involved in the examination of child sexual abuse cases?

Just as in physical abuse the examination should be performed in a child-friendly environment by a doctor who is experienced in dealing with children. There is the need for some hospital-type facilities and a Children's Centre provides a homely environment with these facilities.

The Cleveland affair has left the impression that there is a mystique surrounding the examination in cases of sexual abuse. This should not be the case and it should be seen as part of an ordinary history taking and examination in children where there is concern.

In such children generally the sex of the examining doctor should be irrelevant, however, she or he should be able to attend Case Conferences and give evidence in court. The number of examinations should be kept to a minimum and if possible on one occasion only.

In older girls vaginal examination may be needed and the doctor involved should be experienced at that.

In most cases there is no need for forensic evidence as the suspected abuse is chronic rather than acute. If forensic evidence is required a police surgeon may need to be involved. Many districts have a system of joint examination between police surgeons and paediatricians in cases of child sexual abuse.

History taking and examination in sexual abuse

- A full history should be taken and the examination of genitalia and anus should be preceded by a general examination.
- Internal examination either rectally or vaginally is rarely needed in child sexual abuse.
- There are no signs that are uniquely diagnostic in sexual abuse.
- Many cases of sexual abuse do not have physical signs. This does not mean that the abuse is any less emotionally damaging however.
- The examination of the anus and genitalia should be left to last.
- Evidence of venereal disease should be looked for and suitable swabs from the anus, vulva, vagina or penis should be taken and tested for gonorrhoea and chlamydia. If the gonococcus is found this is very strong evidence of sexual abuse.

Examination of the anus

The anus may be examined before the vulva. The left lateral position is best. The anus should be inspected for bruising and fissures. Bruising around the anal rim is very suggestive of anal abuse. Fissures may be open or healed depending on the time-scale of the abuse.

The reflex anal dilatation test should be performed. In this test the buttocks are parted for up to 30 seconds. In a positive test the anus opens and the rectum can be seen. Sometimes in severe abuse dilatation is seen immediately the anus is examined. The reflex anal dilatation test is not unique to sexual abuse and may be found in severe constipation. Evidence of constipation should therefore be sought by history and abdominal examination.

Examination of the male genitalia

• There may be bruising around the thighs, genitalia, anus, perineum and buttocks and lower abdomen.
• There may be tears and abrasions to the male genitalia. In particular a torn frenulum of the penis.

Examination of the female genitalia

• The female genitalia can be examined on the left lateral position or in younger girls on the mother's lap facing forwards with the legs gently abducted.
• Swabs should be taken if at all possible under the control of the child.
• There may be tears and abrasions to the female genitalia. The hymen in particular should be examined for tears and irregularities. The hymenal opening in young girls is usually no more than 0.6 cm wide.
• Irregularity of the hymen may also be caused by genital disease. Accidental damage is very rare.
• Reddening of the vulva and minor degrees of vulval discharge are very common in young girls and may be associated with minor degrees of wetting with urine.
• Intercrural intercourse (with the penis between the legs)

rarely causes physical signs. The girl may however feel that there was penetration.

Following on from the medical examination

Children very rarely need to be removed from the family as an emergency in child sexual abuse. In many cases the perpetrator is outside the family. Where the perpetrator is within the family it is much better to persuade that person to leave the home rather than exaggerate problems and the child's sense of guilt by removing that child from the home.

Child sexual abuse victims need considerable counselling and psychological help after the event. They particularly need support if there is a court case. They are now spared giving evidence in front of the perpetrator by the use of a video link.

Case Conferences should be held after sexual abuse just as in other types of abuse.

6 The law and child abuse

The *Children Act* 1989

The *Children Act* 1989 is not just another piece of children's legislation. Numerous Acts of Parliament connected with children were repealed, including the *Children and Young Persons Act* 1969, and court structures changed. The intention was to provide 'a simplified and coherent body of law comprehensible, not only to those operating it but also to those affected by its operation'. The Act aims to achieve a balance between protecting children and having procedures that are fair to parents. The date for implementation was October 1991.

Key principles of the Act

(a) The child's welfare must be the paramount consideration of the court.

(b) There is a concept of parental responsibility which replaces parental rights.

(c) Local Authorities have a new duty to promote the upbringing of children in need by their families so far as is consistent with their welfare.

(d) If children are looked after away from home this should preferably be on a voluntary basis and contact with the parents should be maintained.

(e) The Act prohibits a court from making an order unless it is satisfied that it will positively contribute to the child's welfare.

(f) The Act makes it clear that delay in court proceedings is harmful.

(g) There should be a check list of matters which should be considered in most court hearings.

(h) There should be a greater choice in what decisions are available to the court.

Private law proceedings

In private law proceedings between the parents and other individuals the court should aim for practical and not legalistic remedies under the *Children Act* 1989.

The court can decide the following Private Law Orders:

1. With whom a child should live (Residence Orders)
2. What form of contact a child should have with other people (Contact Orders)
3. Any other particular matter concerning a child (Specific Issue Orders)
4. Anything that should be prohibited from being done in relation to the child (Prohibited Steps Order).

The protection of children

The *Children Act* 1989 aims to achieve a balance between protecting a child from harm and unwarranted intervention in a child's family life.

Under the Act the courts can:

1. Order the removal or retention of a child in an emergency (Emergency Protection Orders)
2. Order the assessment of a child when there is real suspicion of harm (Child Assessment Orders)
3. Order that a child be placed under Local Authority care pending a full investigation and hearing of the proceedings (Interim Care Orders)

4. Order that a child be put under the longer care or supervision of the Local Authority (Care and Supervision Orders)
5. Make private law orders concerning the child (Residence Orders, Contact Orders, Specific Issue Orders, Prohibited Steps Orders).

The emergency protection of children

Under the *Children and Young Persons Act* 1969 children could be removed by:

• Place of Safety Orders made by application to a magistrate usually by an officer of the local Social Services Department or by the NSPCC. Place of Safety Orders lasted for up to 28 days. Place of Safety Orders lasting up to 48 hours can be made by the police.

Under the *Children Act* 1989 Place of Safety Orders have been replaced by:

• Emergency Protection Orders which will last for up to eight days. The applicant can apply once for a further seven days. Emergency Protection Orders can be challenged after 72 hours. Applications are made either by an officer of the local Social Services Department or the NSPCC.

The court must be satisfied that there is reasonable cause to believe that the child is likely to suffer significant harm if he or she is not removed to accommodation provided by the applicant or there is reasonable cause to suspect that the child is suffering or is likely to suffer significant harm or that access to the child is denied and is required as a matter of urgency.

In the majority of cases children can be removed to hospital or another suitable place with the voluntary agreement of the parents and orders are not needed.

Under the *Children Act* 1989 the police have the power to remove children to 'police protection' for up to 72 hours where the constable has reasonable cause to believe that the child is likely to suffer significant harm.

• Child Assessment Orders which enable the assessment of a child's health and welfare where concern exists but there is doubt whether emergency action is justified. Only the NSPCC or the Local Authority can apply and the grounds are that the applicant believes the child is suffering or is likely to suffer significant harm and an assessment is unlikely to be allowed without an Order. At the present time it is difficult to know how major a part the Child Assessment Order will play in child protection.

Care proceedings

Under the *Children and Young Persons Act* 1969 care proceedings needed two stages: proof and disposition. Under the *Children Act* 1989 Care Proceedings are one stage and simpler. The court may make a Care Order or a Supervision Order if the child concerned is:

(a) Suffering or is likely to suffer significant harm and
(b) That harm, or likelihood of harm, is attributable to
  i. The standard of care being below what could reasonably be expected or
  ii. The child is beyond parental control.

Care Orders

Care Orders place the care and control of the child with the Local Authority. Sometimes children are placed in foster homes, sometimes in children's homes and sometimes the child is allowed home with the parent(s) whilst remaining under the care of the Local Authority. This is not done until after a Case Conference and all interested parties have been consulted. A contract is usually drawn up between the Social Services Department and the parents.

Supervision Orders

Supervision Orders place the care and control of the child with the parents but give the Local Authority the right to visit that child and supervise their management. This again is often done with a contract.

Interim Care Orders

Interim Care Orders place the care and control of the child with the Local Authority whilst investigations are proceeding and the case for a Care Order is being prepared.

Education Supervision Orders

These orders are made by application by the Local Education Authority (see Chapter 10 on Education, p. 67). The *Children Act* 1989 no longer gives the courts the ability to grant Care Orders on educational grounds alone.

Which courts are involved?

The majority of cases are dealt with by the Magistrates Court. A number of judges are particularly trained in child-care matters and if care proceedings are thought by the local Magistrates' clerk to be particularly complex they are referred on to such a judge in the County Court. Before the implementation of the *Children Act* 1989 complicated cases were often dealt with by the High Court making the child or children concerned Wards of Court. This is not now available to Local Authorities directly although complicated cases may be dealt with by the High Court by referral from lower courts.

Criminal proceedings

In addition to care proceedings there is the separate question of criminal proceedings against the person or persons who have abused children. Charges may be brought for actual bodily harm, grievous bodily harm, child neglect, incest etc. These cases are heard either in the Magistrates Court or in more serious cases the Crown Court.

It used to be thought that the criminal case had no relevance to the care of the child. In practice however it usually makes the protection of that child through the courts much easier. It is the doctor's duty to cooperate with the police and the Crown Prosecution Service in such cases.

Preparing and giving evidence in court

Giving evidence in court is never easy. What appear to be the simplest cases can cause difficulty. The key to success is good preparation.

Preparation

It can often be many months after the initial examination when evidence has to be given in court. Therefore, adequate notes with bruises accurately measured and noted on a topographical chart are essential. In many cases photographs are most important, however, in some cases of fading bruises they can be unimpressive.

Solicitors acting for the Local Authority or those acting for the child or parents often ask you to prepare a report. These reports give an opportunity to marshal all the facts about the case before giving evidence. It is important to state your qualifications and experience as a preamble to the facts of the case and your opinion. Do not give opinions on matters on which you are not experienced. The use of a word processor is invaluable when preparing reports.

It is very often valuable to discuss the evidence you are going to give with the lawyers before the case. This may involve a discussion on the telephone with the solicitor acting for the Local Authority or a more formal conference with counsel arranged by the Crown Prosecution Service.

Police statements

The police sometimes ask doctors to give statements on a case. This can be done by the officer writing down what you say or by writing yourself. A time-saving method can involve having a template for the necessary legal preamble saved on the word processor and then insert after it the report you have already prepared. Such a preamble is shown in Fig. 6.1.

STATEMENT OF WITNESS

(*Criminal Justice Act* 1967, S9; *Magistrates Court Act* 1980, S102; Magistrates Courts Rules 1981, r.70)

STATEMENT OF	Dr First Name Surname
Age of Witness	Over 21
Occupation of Witness	Consultant Paediatrician
Address	Any Hospital, Any town, Any county
	Tel. No. 0000 000000

This statement (consisting of one page each signed by me) is true to the best of my knowledge and belief and I make it knowing that, if it is tendered in evidence, I shall be liable to prosecution if I have wilfully stated in it anything which I know to be false or do not believe to be true.

Dated this 17th Day in October 1990

Signature⎯⎯⎯⎯⎯⎯⎯⎯⎯⎯⎯⎯⎯⎯⎯⎯⎯

Signature Witnessed by⎯⎯⎯⎯⎯⎯⎯⎯⎯⎯⎯⎯⎯⎯⎯

I am a Consultant Paediatrician working for the Any county Health Authority since 1978. I have a special interest in child abuse and have been dealing with the health problems of children for 20 years.

Fig. 6.1   A witness statement

Going to court

The timetable for legal work and medical work is very different. It is very easy to have to spend a great period of time outside the court in child abuse cases waiting to give evidence. Discussion with the lawyers involved in a case is very useful. Often a time for attendance or some way of contact before you are needed in the case can be agreed.

In the witness box

It is important to give the evidence that you are going to give clearly and slowly. When asked for your qualifications and experience give all the degrees you have, how long you have been dealing with children and what experience you have of child abuse. Do not attempt to be an expert on things you are not.

Lawyers often try to get you to assess bruises and other injuries individually. Try very hard not to go along this road and say that in such cases you have to consider the whole examination not individual injuries.

7 The sudden infant death syndrome

Sudden infant death syndrome (SIDS), when a baby dies unexpectedly in the first months of life without an obvious cause, is one of the most distressing events that can ever happen to a family. It is now the most common cause of death in the first year of life after the neonatal period. The paediatrician should be involved in:

● Counselling and helping the parents after the death
● Trying to prevent a further recurrence in the family
● Trying to reduce the incidence in the population as a whole

Why should children die from sudden infant death syndrome?

The question of why children should die from SIDS is an intriguing one and one to which we do not have the whole answer. We do know that there are a number of clues in the epidemiology of SIDS that make a single factor such as a conduction defect of the heart, cow's milk allergy or a metabolic defect most unlikely. We know that the maximum incidence of SIDS is in the winter months and that the total mortality decreases with age and is at a maximum between 2 and 4 months. We also know that SIDS is more common in poorer families, in young and single mothers and at the weekend. Minor symptoms such as a mild cough or cold sometimes precede the death of a child from SIDS. It does seem that in most cases the mode of death is a respiratory one.

There has been evidence to suggest that SIDS is rare in some societies such as in Hong Kong. It may be that there is something in fundamental child-care practices that is protective against SIDS. Certainly SIDS is rare where children are kept close to adults and observed all the time.

There is an increasing volume of work that suggests that a number of significant factors are commoner in SIDS victims than controls. These are:

- The baby lying prone on its abdomen rather than supine on its back or on its side.
- The baby having thick quilts, duvets or blankets
- Parental smoking

Counselling and helping parents after they have lost a baby from the sudden infant death syndrome

The effect of having a baby die of SIDS is devastating for the whole family. It is made more difficult because as a sudden unexplained death it has to be reported to the Coroner and investigated by the Coroner's officer, a policeman. It is very important that an experienced person counsels parents who have lost a baby in this way as soon as possible after the death. A paediatrician is in an ideal position to do this. A booklet is available for parents whose child has died from SIDS from:

The Foundation for the Study of Infant Deaths
35 Belgrave Square
London SW1X 8PS

Telephone 071-235 1721 Cot Death enquiries
          071-235 0965 general enquiries

The people who counsel the parents will need to mention:

- The role of the Coroner and that the Coroner's officer, a policeman, will need to be involved
- That the baby's death will need to be registered
- That either a burial or cremation can be chosen
- That they can see the baby again
- Why the baby died and what is SIDS
- That it was not anybody's fault
- How brothers and sisters deal with the problem
- How to deal with grief, i.e. that it is a natural and healthy thing and should not be suppressed.

Preventing cases of the sudden infant death syndrome in the community

As SIDS is more common in vulnerable families, there is some evidence that it can be prevented by placing community child health resources, such as health visitors, selectively in these families. In particular, minor illness in babies should be dealt with efficiently and quickly.

There are certain practical steps that all parents can be told about as part of the Child Surveillance Programme. These are:

- Lying the baby on its side or back not its front
- Not allowing the baby to become overheated by using duvets, too many blankets etc
- Not smoking
- Pertussis immunization (pertussis may sometimes be associated with SIDS)
- Encouraging breast feeding

Preventing cases of the sudden infant death syndrome in siblings

Parents are always very concerned in those situations. A happy medium needs to be struck between this natural concern and overanxiety. Clearly the advice for any parent particularly is relevant here. All parents in this situation need to be counselled. Good antenatal care is also important.

Most parents ask for apnoea monitors and they may be reassuring for them. There is no evidence, however, that they prevent recurrences of SIDS. They need servicing regularly.

8 Prevention of accidents

Accidents are an important problem in childhood. They are the most common cause of death in children over the age of 1 year in Britain. In 1990, 616 children under 14 years of age died in England and Wales from accidents. Nearly twice as many children between 5 and 14 years died from accidents than from malignant disease (71 compared to 37 children per million). Accidents account for about a third of deaths of children between the ages of 1 and 14 years.

Accidents also cause significant handicap and suffering to children. Children may be brain damaged following head injury, near drowning or suffocation episodes. Cosmetic damage following burns, scalds and road traffic accidents may be very damaging psychologically to the child.

Prevention of accidents

The prevention of accidents to children is therefore being increasingly recognized as an important part of the role of a community paediatrician. Doctors who treat children and see the effects of their accidents are in a unique position in society to alert the community to the problem and to take action to prevent accidents. What is more difficult is how this is to be achieved.

It is very tempting to think that all that is needed is to

alert the public to the dangers of accidents to children by educational campaigns. The evidence that these are effective, however, is unconvincing. It is also tempting to look on accidents to children as a whole and think of general solutions to the problem. All the evidence, however, suggests that accidents to children have been prevented by looking at an individual type of accident, looking at the detailed epidemiology of that accident, and evaluating a solution before its widespread introduction. In almost all the cases where accident prevention solutions have been shown to be effective those solutions have been ones that involve environmental change rather than education.

Road traffic accidents

Road traffic accidents (RTAs) are the most common cause of accidental deaths in childhood. Their prevention remains a major challenge. In 1990, 328 children died from RTAs in England and Wales. Road traffic accidents are also a major cause of long-term disability.

Pedestrian road traffic accidents

Pedestrian RTAs are most common in children from socially deprived families living in an environment where they are not separated from traffic. Poor families are also often under considerable stress. Boys between the ages of 5 and 8 years are at maximum risk from RTAs particularly after school. They are unable to estimate the speed or dangers of traffic and to foresee dangerous situations.

Safety and traffic education are unlikely to prevent RTAs by themselves. Kerb drill is not perceived by young children to detect traffic and is not thought sufficient by itself to ward off the dangers of the road. Adequate explanations of exactly what is involved in road safety are given by very few children. In Britain it has been suggested that the Green Cross Code prevented accidents when it was introduced, however, careful analysis of the figures suggests this was not the case.

Pedestrian RTAs can be prevented by modification of the environment. This can be done by redesigning roads in residential areas to give priority to pedestrians and to separate them from traffic. The speed of traffic can be reduced by speed bumps and other traffic calming measures and play areas can be provided keeping children off dangerous streets.

Accidents to child passengers in cars

Unrestrained children become 'missiles' inside cars during even quite low velocity crashes. There is good evidence that child restraint systems also prevent injury and death. They also improve child behaviour. It is now the law in Britain that if seat belts are fitted to the rear of a car it is the driver's legal responsibility to ensure that children use them. Encouraging parents to obey the law and carry children in cars in approved restraints should form part of a child surveillance programme.

Which restraint system to use?

Babies are now best carried in a special portable infant carrier which is usually rear-facing.

A carry cot held by straps is an alternative but the cot and not the baby directly is restrained.

Children between 10 and 18 kilogrammes should have a child car seat. They can either be fixed directly to the car by two- or four-point anchorage or be fitted with adult seat belts whichever is particularly convenient. For children between 18 and 36 kilogrammes adult seat belts should be used with a booster cushion.

Bicycle accidents to children

Parents should be encouraged to give thought to the type of bicycle they buy for their child and to the proper maintenance of the chain, gears and brakes. Bicycle training for children also seems sensible. There are factors in bicycle design which are important to safety. The majority of severe injuries that children receive are those to the head. A boy has a 1 in

80 chance of having a bicycle head injury severe enough for admission to hospital in childhood. Cycle helmets are a logical solution to this problem and are becoming more easily available and used more often.

Checklist for health care professionals to prevent road traffic accidents to children

• Encourage parents of children 8 years old and under to take them to school.
• Encourage councils to develop schemes to separate children from traffic.
• Encourage councils to provide play areas for children. Particularly in inner city areas.
• Encourage local action in dealing with dangerous road situations, particularly near schools.
• Encourage the use of car safety seats for children and acceptance of the law. Encourage the use of loan schemes and first ride safe ride schemes.
• Encourage the use of bicycle safety helmets.
• Encourage parents to let their children attend bicycle riding instruction and to maintain the bicycles adequately.

Burns and scalds in children

More children die accidentally from burns and scalds than any other cause apart from road traffic accidents. The majority of the children who die do so in house fires. Many children under the age of 5 years are scarred for life from scalds. This happens most commonly from hot fluids from a cup or a mug, but significant numbers are scalded from teapots, kettles and in baths. Children are also burnt from small igniting sources such as matches, from out-door fires, from space heating and from cooking equipment.

Burn and scald accidents to children are most common in disadvantaged families who often live in an environment where smoking is common, where there are open fires and where there is inflammable furniture. They are also under psycho-social stress making supervision of young children difficult.

The prevention of burn and scald accidents to children

There are a number of environmental measures which have helped or would help if introduced in prevention of burn and scald injuries in children.

Fires have been or could be prevented by:

Stopping the source of the fire

This can be done by:
- Introducing central heating rather than open fires
- Introducing fireguards
- Reducing smoking
- Banning dangerous fireworks

Reducing the flammability of the child's environment

- Much upholstered furniture produces toxic fumes when it burns. Foam that causes dangerous fumes is now banned.
- The flammability of nightdresses and other clothes should be reduced under the Nightdress (Safety) Regulations 1967.

Providing a warning if a fire takes place

- Smoke detectors are widely used in the USA and are becoming more established in Britain. They have an important role in the prevention of conflagrations and their use should be encouraged both in public and private housing.

The prevention of scalds in children is a difficult problem. A wider use of mugs and the elimination of unstable cups is to be encouraged. A number of children injure themselves with spillage from kettles and these injuries can be avoided by the use of coil or sprung electric kettle flexes without large expense. Some children scald themselves by pulling saucepans down from cookers. Many of these incidents can be prevented by reducing access to the cooker and by cooker guards.

Checklist for health care professionals to prevent burn and scald accidents to children

- Encourage the disposal of dangerous foam furniture.
- Encourage the use of smoke alarms both by individuals and by local councils.

- Discourage open fires. If they have to be used then use fireguards.
- Emphasize the dangers of hot liquids.
- Place kitchen units on either side of the cooker or fit a cooker guard.
- Use coiled flex electric kettles.
- Encourage the safe use of fireworks.

Drowning and near drowning in childhood

Drowning is the third most common cause of accidental death in children in the UK. Near drowning is unusual as, unlike most other accidents, it is an infrequent cause of presentation to the Accident and Emergency Department. Some children survive near drowning episodes and are left seriously handicapped although many children also survive prolonged immersion neurologically normal.

Where do children drown and how can they be prevented from doing so?

Drowning deaths and near-drowning incidents in childhood can be divided into clear types with definite separate age ranges and epidemiology. Each site of drowning therefore has separate preventive measures that could be applied.

Bath drownings

Age range: Babies and toddlers

Special features: Families of low socioeconomic class and highly mobile. Child abuse should always be considered.

Prevention: As part of the programme of child surveillance.

Garden pond drownings

Age range: Under fives

Special features: Children can drown in quite small shallow ponds. The commonest story is of an unsupervised toddler wandering off when visiting friends or relatives.

Prevention: Fence ponds, especially in parks and garden centres. A grid just under the water can prevent children being able to immerse themselves. As part of the programme of child surveillance.

Private swimming pool drownings

Age range: Under fives

Special features: Children wander off unsupervised and either fall into the pool or crawl under the covers. It is much more common than public pool drowning.

Prevention: Fencing which prevents children from having access to private pools with self-shutting gates.

Public pool drownings

Age range: Over fives

Special features: Many children go swimming but very few drown since supervision has improved.

Prevention: Good supervision with use of Health and Safety Regulations.

River, canal and lake drownings

Age range: Older boys

Special features: Boys play unsupervised and get into trouble in deep water. Many are non-swimmers.

Prevention: Discourage unsupervised swimming. Teach children to swim.

Sea drownings

Age range: All ages

Special features: It is not a major problem, only six children died in the UK from sea drownings in 1988.

Prevention: Teach children to swim. Use life jackets and buoyancy aids.

Checklist for health care professionals to prevent drowning accidents to children

● Advise parents to fence off private pools, to take care with pool cover design and to drain pools in winter.
● Ensure swimming is adequately supervised especially in non-municipal public pools (i.e. holiday camps) and at lakes such as those in country parks.
● Advise parents to teach their children to swim.
● Advise parents regarding the dangers to young children in baths and in garden ponds.
● Advise parents to fence off, grid or remove garden ponds.
● Ensure life jackets and buoyancy aids are available for children in boats.

Architectural accidents and falls in children

The design of homes where children live is important for their safety. Many falls, accidents with glass and burns can be prevented by good design. Making homes safer for children should be an essential part of a child surveillance programme.

Falls in childhood

Falls are the commonest cause of presentation to the Accident and Emergency Department.
    Falls can be on one level, for example:

● Falling on the pavement
● Falling at home
● Falling in the school playground

Falls can also be from one level to another:

● Falling from furniture
● Falling down the stairs – prevented by better design and stair-gates

- Falling from toys
- Falling from baby walkers which are potentially dangerous
- Falling from windows – prevented by using safety catches or window guards
- Falling from cliffs and mountains
- Falling from play equipment

Glass injuries

Children who fall through glass can sustain severe lacerations which may cause blood loss, scarring and injury to arteries, nerves and tendons. There may also be internal injuries.

Most glass injuries in childhood can be prevented by the use of safety glazing, for example:

- Laminated safety glass absorbs impact and is resistant to penetration. Laminated glass is only about 1.8 times more expensive than annealed flat glass.
- Plastic safety film can also be used on existing glazing.

Finding unsafe glass and suggesting safer alternatives whilst visiting the home should be part of a child surveillance programme.

Checklist for health care professionals to prevent architectural accidents and falls to children

- Check the design of stairs for child safety.
- Advise parents to use stair gates if there are toddlers in house.
- Advise parents against baby walkers.
- Check window and balcony designs for child safety. Advise the use of catches if necessary.
- Advise the use of safety glass or safety film for low level glazing.

Accidents to children at play and recreation

Playground injuries

Playgrounds are dangerous places for children. It has been estimated that there are 24 000 such accidents each year in England and Wales. These accidents can be prevented by attention to safe design.

Surface of the playground

Replace concrete with an impact-absorbing surface such as a granular bark compound or a specially prepared, rubberized surface.

Swings

Reduce impact injuries by making swing seats of an impact-absorbing substance, indeed, even an old tyre will suffice. Fence off swings to prevent children rushing into them.

Slides

Replace the old-fashioned types where children climb a ladder to a platform far from the ground with a slide that follows a contour of a hill – children receive a much smaller fall if a mishap occurs.

Climbing frames

Reduce the height. It is just as much fun playing horizontally as vertically, and it is much less far to fall. Impact-absorbing surfaces will also reduce injuries with climbing frames.

Roundabouts

Replace types such as the 'Witches Hat' which can cause falls and trap limbs.

Preventing sports injuries

All forms of sport and recreation have some risk and every year children are injured and a few die during sports and leisure activities. Children cannot be protected from all risks in recreational activity, which are important in the development of personality and in physical development. On the other hand, children should not be exposed to unnecessary risk. Risks can be reduced by sensible supervision and other safety measures, for example:

● Hill and mountain climbing expeditions need careful supervision by experienced guides and teachers.
● Rugby football neck injuries and paraplegia can be reduced if teams are not of different ages and ability, and referees can also pay particular attention to collapsing the scrum and to mauls after tackles.
● Horse riding needs good head protection to prevent head injury. Many traditional riding hats offered little protection for the rider. In April 1984, a new British Standard, BS 6473, for protective hats for riders was introduced.

Dog bites

Dog bites to children are very common with 1 in a 100 children a year presenting to the Accident and Emergency Department with this problem. Many of the accidents occur in the home, or with dogs well known to the children. A significant number of children are bitten, however, in public areas, particularly play areas. The majority of dog bites are minor, but severe lacerations, particularly facial lacerations, do occur. Parents should be informed of the dangers of dogs as part of a child surveillance programme. Small children should always be supervised when they are around dogs including family pets.

Checklist for health care professionals to prevent recreational accidents to children

● Find playgrounds in the district and check on design and surfaces. Investigate any playground injuries.
● Influence safe design with local councils and accident committees. Campaign if necessary.
● Be aware of the dangers of dogs as part of a health visitor's accident prevention package.

- Keep dogs out of playgrounds.
- Ensure sporting activities for children are supervised.
- Ensure teams are of a similar age and ability.
- Ensure horse riding is well taught.
- Ensure head protection for horse riding is worn and is to British Standard, BS 6473.

Poisoning in children

There are several types of poisoning seen in childhood:

- Accidental child poisoning
- Deliberate self-poisoning in older children
- Non-accidental poisoning
- Iatrogenic poisoning

Accidental child poisoning

Accidental poisoning is predominantly seen in children under the age of 5 years with a peak age for children of 30 months. A very few children die from poisoning each year but many more are admitted to hospital for treatment and observation. Still more present to hospital Accident and Emergency Departments, with as many as 19% of children having had at least one previous incident of poisoning or suspected poisoning. It seems strange that young children may wish to take poisons. It does not seem that availability of the poison is a factor but more a child's reaction to family psycho-social stress such as family illness or a move. 'Hyperactive' children are also more liable to take poisons.

Preventing accidental child poisoning

Educational campaigns have not been successful in preventing accidental child poisoning. Families under stress are unlikely to remember safety propaganda.

Child-resistant containers (CRCs), which prevent the toddler from getting at the potential poison, have proved successful when evaluated in a community in the USA, and have been introduced into the USA and UK. In the UK they are now used by regulation on paracetamol and salicylate preparations and on certain household products such as white spirit. Their use is a professional requirement for pharmacists. Opaque blister packs are an alternative.

Poison Line: London – Guy's Hospital. Telephone 071-955 5095
               Edinburgh – Royal Infirmary. Telephone 031-229 2477
               Cardiff – Llandough Hospital. Telephone 0222 709901
               Belfast – Royal Victoria Infirmary. Telephone 0232 240503

Checklist for health care professionals to prevent accidental poisoning in children

● Encourage the use of child-resistant caps by pharmacists. Discourage prescribing of quinine and barbiturates etc.
● Encourage the storage of medicines and household products away from the reach of children.

Checklist for health care professionals to prevent accidents to children

● Obtain accurate accident statistics for the district
● Form a local accident committee
● Establish links with councillors, parents' organizations etc.
● Deal with each accident individually
● Establish a checklist and programme of surveillance and prevention for health care professionals

(Reproduced from Sibert, J.R., 1991, *Arch Dis Child*, **66**, 890–3.)

9 Adoption and fostering

Although the number of babies available for adoption is now relatively small, more older children need to be adopted now than before. Many of these children have been subject to child abuse or may have special needs.

Adoption and fostering are under the control of adoption agencies whose work is under the strict control of the law. All County Councils, London Boroughs and Metropolitan Boroughs have their own adoption agency. In addition to this there are adoption societies such as The Catholic Children Society, The Children's Society, National Children's Home, Barnardos etc. who work separately from local authorities. Lists of adoption agencies can be obtained from the:

British Agencies for Adoption and Fostering
11 Southwark Street
London SE1 1RQ

Why do people adopt?

Many people who adopt cannot have children themselves, however, it takes time to come to terms with infertility and it may not be a good idea for couples to rush into adoption. Some people just want to add to their family.

Adoption in practice

The adoption of a child is guided by three principles:

1. Is the adoption in this child's best interests?
2. Is adoption appropriate for these applicants?
3. Are these particular applicants suitable for this particular child?

In the past many people felt that they wanted to adopt babies, however, fewer and fewer babies are available for adoption. It may be easier for those of Afro-Caribbean, African or Asian descent to be able to adopt babies.

Most adoption agencies expect couples to be married for at least three years before they adopt and to have had infertility tests. Couples need to be at least 21 years of age to adopt by law, and most adoption agencies expect couples to be in their late twenties or early thirties.

There is a special situation with step-parents who wish to adopt children, one that may be limited by new adoption regulations.

Many people now adopt older children. These are children either with special needs or children who have been in care for a period of time. There are clearly particular problems adopting a child from a different ethnic and cultural group and on the whole adoption agencies wish to make certain that children go to families of the same ethnic origin. This may not be possible in all cases.

To adopt a child an Adoption Order is needed. These are usually applied for when the child has been with prospective adoptive parents for at least three months. Adoption agencies usually wish for a rather longer period of time.

Intercountry adoption

The principles of adoption may be difficult to apply in these situations, in particular what are the child's best interests. The subject is discussed by the *Social Services Inspectorate Document CI(90) 17*. There are certain principles that apply:

• All intercountry adoptions should be through competent authorities and the relevant documents should be available. The laws of the country should be respected.
• All applications should be subject to standards equivalent to those operating in the UK.
• It should be established before a child leaves its country that there are parents for him or her in the UK.
• There should be adequate counselling for those involved.
• The legal validity of the adoption should be assured.

Racial considerations in adoption and fostering

It is considered good practice in adoption and fostering for children to be placed in families of a similar racial background to themselves. This is because children who are placed in families of different race suffer increased problems with their identity as they grow up.

Although there are of course many successful transracial adoptions, adoption agencies try to find suitable foster and adoptive families from ethnic minorities. Problems arise because there may not be enough foster families from particular racial groups in an emergency. Children may therefore be bonded to their foster family and change may be more damaging to the child than being brought up in a family of a different race. Doctors should take a pragmatic approach to advice they give on such matters.

The doctor's role in adoption and fostering

Doctors dealing with children have an important part to play in the adoption and fostering of children. They advise adoption agencies on the medical aspect of children to be adopted or fostered and they may also advise agencies on the suitability of couples for adopting or fostering children.

Doctors dealing with children in care may also take a lead role in the decision to go to court to free a child for adoption.

The British Agencies for Adoption and Fostering provides

a useful source of advice for doctors. Anybody dealing frequently with adoption issues would be well advised to join this organization.

The *Adoption Agency Regulations* 1983

The *Adoption Agency Regulations* 1983 in England and Wales came to force in 1984 and gave statutory recognition to existing good practice. Each adoption agency now has a statutory duty to nominate at least one registered medical practitioner as the agency's medical advisor. It is possible to have one solo medical advisor who deals with both paediatrics and general medicine, and gives advice about the child and the prospective adoptive parents. It is also possible to have a number of medical advisors with particular interests. It may be also that a solo medical advisor will obtain advice from other doctors. Such a person should be a member of the Adoption Panel and will collect medical information.

A medical advisor should be involved by the Agency in the following statutory duties:

● Providing the prospective adopters with written information about the child's health history and current state of health.
● Sending, before placement, a written report on the child's health history and current state of health to prospective adopters' registered medical practitioner, usually the GP.
● Notifying, before placement, the District Health Authority in the area in which the prospective adopter resides.
● Notifying, before placement, the Local Authority, Social Services and Local Education Authority in the area in which the prospective adopter resides if the child is considered by the medical advisor to be handicapped or to have special educational needs.

After adoption

It is important that adoption should be discussed quite naturally right from the start. At any time from the age of 18 years adopted children have a right to their original birth certificate if they want it, although their adoptive parents may have already given it to them. Adoption agencies always try and help adoptive parents with this process.

Fostering

Foster parents are clearly very important for children in the care of the Local Authority. Although it is not the same as adoption it is a very important service for the child. Allowances are paid which are meant to cover the costs of fostering. Some children start off being fostered for a short-term and then end up being fostered long-term.

10 Education

Children over the age of 5 years spend a great deal of their time at school and therefore their education is clearly a vital part of their life and upbringing. Any assessment of a child in a hospital or community setting should include information on the child's education.

In England and Wales education is the responsibility of County Councils with the inspectorate and policy coming from the Department of Education and Science in England or the Welsh Office.

School not only provides education, but also provides a background where children can learn to relate to their peers. It is this aspect of schooling that children most miss out on if they do not attend regularly. It is very difficult to regain time missed. One of the key aims of doctors concerned with child health is to ensure that children are able to go to school.

Getting information on a child's education

Having said how important it is to find out how children are getting on at school, it is sometimes difficult for doctors to actually obtain that information. This information can be obtained from:

- *Parents:* It is always important to ask about a child's

educational progress when talking to parents. It is also important to recognize that the information given may not be accurate.

● *Teachers in the school:* It may be more accurate directly to ask the school. However, sometimes teachers are unwilling to discuss children's progress with doctors that they do not know.

● *Teachers in the hospital:* The hospital school teacher is an important liaison person with teachers in schools in the community. They are able to talk to teachers on a teacher-to-teacher basis, which is often very valuable. This method also has the benefit of speed.

● *School Nurses:* The School Nurse has a key role in many districts and will often be able to give valuable information quickly.

● *The school doctor:* This method has the ability of focusing directly on medical problems, but may have considerable delays within it.

● *Educational psychologists:* The School Psychological Service will often be able to give direct information on children who have been referred to them for assessment.

● *Educational welfare officers:* Information on school attendance is available from educational welfare officers, and also the action that they have taken regarding non-attendance at school.

What information can be obtained from the school?

Information can be obtained on:

● A child's general progress in school and whether he or she is keeping up with his or her peers.
● The child's educational attainment level.
● The child's attendance record.
● Whether a child has any behavioural problems at school.
● Whether a child has had any special tests on their educational ability.
● Whether a child has problems with bullying or relating to individual children.
● Whether a child is able to participate in school games.
● Whether a child's friendships are satisfactory.

It may be that relatively trivial breakdowns of relationships between children can cause great concern and non-organic problems.

Influencing a child's education

If there are specific problems at school it is probably best to talk to the head teacher in primary schools or to the year tutor in secondary schools. If this proves impossible then the community health doctor concerned with that school may be able to deal with the problem directly.

If there are continuing problems it may be necessary to write to or telephone the Director of Education at the County Council, London or Metropolitan Borough.

In some cases it may be appropriate to talk with or write to a school governor or the local councillor. These names can be obtained from the Council.

Educational psychologists often need to be involved with children where there is concern regarding their educational progress. The child can be referred directly or there can again be a discussion with the teachers.

It is important to recognize those children who are under-achieving for their intelligence level.

Recognizing medical problems at school

Medical conditions that may retard a child's education

There are a number of clear medical problems that may affect a child's education that may not be immediately obvious. These include:

- Deafness
- Epilepsy
- Visual problems
- Behavioural problems

Dyslexia and specific learning difficulties at school

Dyslexia is a specific learning difficulty that results in problems with reading, spelling, written prose and sometimes arithmetic. There may be a family history of such difficulties. The word 'dyslexia' is a controversial one and there have been considerable arguments in medical, psychological and educational circles about its use. Nevertheless, there is a definite proportion of children who have a reading age which is significantly below that expected from their chronological age and their IQ. Such children, who may be described as having dyslexia, often also have:

- A disorder of language function
- A disorder of visual perception
- A disorder of coordination

The diagnosis of dyslexia is essentially one for the teacher and the educational psychologist. However, children may present with emotional and non-organic problems. Other physical problems such as hearing or vision problems should be excluded. The occupational therapist may well be able to help with coordination problems.

A child's poor performance at school may cause great anxiety to parents. Dyslexia may be thought of as one of the causes of this poor performance which may not necessarily be the case. Doctors may be asked to advise in this situation. The approach should be a multidisciplinary one recognizing the key role of teachers.

The school health service

It used to be standard practice that all children should be medically examined on school entry. Many people now believe that this is not necessary and that a school health review with selective examinations can be safely undertaken leaving more time for responding to the problems of teachers and recognizing children with special needs. The school nurse should have a key role in this process.

This is a subject of considerable controversy, however, where the general practice is good and community health records are adequate a selective medical system and school entry health review is satisfactory. All children should have hearing, vision and growth assessed on school entry.

Children with special educational needs

What special education is available?

Following the Warnock Committee Report, the *Education Act* 1981 recommended that children should, if at all possible, be educated in normal schools. It should be the aim of health care professionals working with children to facilitate this as much as possible.

However, there are some circumstances where children do need special educational help. The types of schools that may be involved are:

- Schools for children with physical handicaps
- Schools for children with moderate learning difficulties
- Schools for children with severe learning difficulties
- Schools for children with hearing impairments
- Schools for visually handicapped children
- Schools for children with speech and language delay
- Schools for children with behavioural problems

Often integration can be achieved at least partly by special classes in ordinary schools.

Identification of children with special educational needs

Under the *Education Act* 1981 if doctors or other health authority staff know of a child over 2 years of age who is likely to have educational special needs they should inform the Local Education Authority (LEA) after discussion and permission from the parents. Information of course may come to the LEA from other sources such as the nursery or school.

The LEA may then decide to issue a statement under Section 5 of the Act.

Assessment of children with educational special needs

Under the *Education Act* 1981, the LEA must seek educational, medical and psychological advice on children in every case when an assessment is made under Section 5 of the Act. The Act aims to provide a common approach to advice for children with special educational needs. A report should aim to:

- Provide a diagnosis
- Give the relevant aspects of the child's functioning including strengths and weakness
- Assess the child's relationship to the environment at home and school
- Record the child's past history
- Establish which provision should be made for the child to develop independence
- Recommend facilities and resources to promote these aims (but without naming a specific educational provision)

There should be a medical officer designated in each district to coordinate information on children with special educational needs. He or she should coordinate and collect information from doctors and specialized support services such as speech therapists, occupational therapists and physiotherapists.

After the LEA has obtained information from all the professionals concerned (including a detailed report from the educational psychologist) a Statement of Educational Need is then prepared and sent to the parents. If they accept (they have 30 days to appeal) a school which takes into account the child's educational need will be nominated by the local education department.

Under the *Education Act* 1981 LEAs should review statements on an annual basis. If this review reveals there has been a significant change in the circumstances of the child a reassessment is made and a new statement issued.

Home tuition

Home tuition is sometimes put forward as an alternative to school, however, it is very seldom for more than a few hours a week. It does not really provide an adequate basis for the child's needs, particularly those of social contact with other children. It should be avoided if possible. In particular it should not be used in cases of non-organic illness and school refusal.

There may be children with severe chronic illness, such as oncological patients and those with chronic renal failure and cystic fibrosis, where home tuition is unavoidable for short periods. Doctors will often be asked to advise on this.

11 Immunization

The standard immunization schedule

The Department of Health and the Welsh Office have a standard immunization schedule which is recommended by the Joint Committee on Vaccination and Immunization. This schedule involves immunizing babies against diphtheria, tetanus, pertussis (D/T/P) and polio; infants against measles, mumps, rubella (MMR); providing booster diptheria, tetanus (D/T) and polio at school entry; immunizing teenage girls against rubella; and all teenagers against BCG and with booster tetanus and polio.

The emphasis of the immunization programme has gone from the community to the general practice situation with tight immunization percentages in the audit mechanisms of the GP contract.

The standard immunization schedule is changed from time to time. The last change was in May 1990.

The immunization schedule

D/P/T and oral polio (primary course):
    1st dose – at 2 months
    2nd dose – at 3 months
    3rd dose – at 4 months

MMR:

At 12–18 months (it can be given at any age over 12 months)

D/T and oral polio booster and MMR (if not already done):

At school entry (4–5 years)

Rubella (girls only) and BCG:

At 10–14 years (with 3 weeks between BCG and rubella)

Booster tetanus and oral polio:

At 15–18 years.

The major change to the previous schedule has been the accelerated D/T/P and polio immunizations. This:

• Fits in with the World Health Organization Recommendations
• Gives earlier protection against pertussis
• Gives the opportunity to give combined immunization with child surveillance
• Gives fewer opportunities for postponement due to minor illnesses

Route of administration

Oral polio vaccine must never be injected. All the other immunizations except BCG are given by deep subcutaneous or intramuscular injection. BCG is given intradermally.

Contraindications against immunizations on the schedule

General

• Immunization is only rarely contraindicated.
• D/T/P and polio should be postponed if there is an acute illness. Minor infections without pyrexia or systemic symptoms are not contraindications to immunization.

Immunization should not be carried out if there has been:

• A previous severe local reaction (induration and redness involving most of the anterolateral part of the thigh or most of the circumference of the upper arm).
• A previous severe systemic reaction (fever more than 39.5°C within 48 hours of the vaccine, anaphylaxis, broncho-spasm, prolonged screaming or convulsions occurring within 72 hours).

Contraindications to specific vaccines on the programme

Pertussis

A family history of allergy is not a contraindication to whooping cough immunization nor are stable neurological conditions such as cerebral palsy and muscular dystrophy.

Children with problem histories such as:

• A documented history of cerebral damage in the neo-natal period
• A personal history of convulsions
• A family history of idiopathic epilepsy

need special consideration. They may be at more risk of convulsions but they are also more at risk of major problems if they get the disease themselves. Many of them can be immunized. If in doubt expert advice from a paediatrician can be obtained.

Poliomyelitis

Diarrhoea and vomiting are contraindications to oral polio-myelitis vaccine. So are high-dose corticosteroids and malig-nant disease.

Measles, mumps, rubella vaccine

Measles, mumps, rubella (MMR) vaccine should be given even if the child is said to have had measles, mumps or rubella in the past. The diagnosis is often difficult and even if it is correct the child needs protecting from the other diseases.

Contraindicated children include:

• Those with malignant disease or altered immunity
• Those with allergies to neomycin or kanomycin

- Those who have been immunized with another live vaccine (i.e. BCG) within the previous 3 weeks
- Those with true egg allergy (i.e. generalized urticaria and anaphylactic reaction, not dislike or refusal to eat eggs)

Rubella

Rubella vaccine should not be given to a woman or girl known to be pregnant. Pregnancy should be avoided for one month after immunization.

BCG immunization

BCG should not be given to children:

- With malignant disease or altered immunity
- On corticosteroids
- With positive sensitivity tests to tuberculin protein (i.e. Mantoux tests, Heaf tests etc.)
- With septic skin conditions
- With a fever

Other immunizations available

Influenza

This vaccine is only recommended in childhood for those children with some chronic disease that would make influenza particularly dangerous. These include:

- Chronic lung disease (such as cystic fibrosis)
- Congenital heart disease
- Chronic renal disease

Hepatitis B

This vaccine should be given to:

- Health care personnel (doctors, nurses, laboratory technicians) who are thought to be at risk
- Patients and family contacts, i.e. those entering institutions for the mentally handicapped, those who might require renal dialysis etc.

- Persons visiting countries of high incidence
- Infants of mothers with hepatitis B

Rabies

The vaccine used at present is the human diploid cell vaccine (HDCV).

It may be used as pre-exposure prophylaxis but it is available for those at occupational risk only on the NHS. Children who are going abroad may be immunized but not free of charge.

It may also be used as post-exposure treatment.

Cholera

Cholera vaccine is of limited use. It is no longer recommended by the WHO for routine use but may still be needed by some countries as an entry requirement.

Typhoid

Monovalent typhoid vaccine is recommended to those travelling abroad apart from Europe, North America, Australia and New Zealand. It is not recommended for those children under one year of age.

The dose is 0.5 ml for children over 10 years of age and adults, and 0.25 ml for children of 1–10 years, 4–6 weeks apart. A booster can be given after 3 years.

Yellow fever

The 17 D virus strain vaccine is recommended for children over 9 months old travelling to infected areas (Tropical Africa and South America). The dose is 0.5 ml.

Others

Vaccines are being introduced for haemophilus influenzae type B and meningococcal disease.

12 Child surveillance

In 1989 the Working Party on Child Health Surveillance (where paediatricians, health visitors and general practitioners were represented) reported and suggested that the pattern of monitoring children in the UK should be changed. A programme was suggested for child health surveillance of what was thought on the best evidence to be effective and worthwhile. As well as the programme of surveillance it was suggested there should be much more listening to parental concerns and much more positive action regarding health. The Working Party purposely did not discuss who should actually undertake the surveillance programme.

The benefits of a surveillance programme should include:

● The formation of a positive relationship which allows positive promotion of health
● Preventive work
● Guidance on important child health topics
● Maintenance of a body of knowledge with the community on child health and development

What should be part of a programme of child health surveillance?

The Working Party found clear indications for examining for the following in a programme of child health surveillance:

- Full physical examination at 6 weeks
- Congenital dislocation of hips
- Undescended testes
- Congenital heart disease
- Growth disorders (including head circumference and weight at 6 weeks and weight and height at the age of 3 years)
- Simple developmental milestones (sitting, walking, talking)
- Hearing defects
- Vision defects
- Behavioural problems
- Screening for phenylketonuria (PKU) and hypothyroidism (these are done on the blood spots collected by community midwife or health visitor)

The Working Party did not find clear indications for examining for the following in a programme of child health surveillance:

- Laboratory tests for muscular dystrophy (CPK estimation) and cystic fibrosis
- Routine examination of the urine
- Haemoglobinopathy in the general population
- Iron deficiency anaemia
- Adolescent scoliosis
- Formal development tests
- Hypertension

Surveillance in certain populations

Child health surveillance may well include special tests in certain situations. These could include:

- Sickle cell anaemia in children of African or West Indian countries
- Thalassaemia in children from Cypriot families and from India and Pakistan
- Iron deficiency anaemia in poorer families
- Echocardiography in children with Down's syndrome

Parent held records

Coming at the same time as the Working Party on Child Health Surveillance a further Working Party discussed professional and parent held records used in child health surveillance.

It is generally now accepted that a set parent held record should be the main document in following children in the first years of life. This gives the opportunity for parents to be much more involved in the care of their children and dealing with problems. It should also prevent duplication of records. Although there may be concerns with child abuse patients these should not be severe enough to cause major problems. In these cases separate records might be held in parallel with those held by the parent.

Health promotion

Health promotion should be a clear part of any programme of child health surveillance. Topics mentioned should include:

- Promotion of breast feeding
- Accident prevention
- Immunization
- Prevention of child abuse
- Dealing with behavioural problems
- Prevention of sudden infant death syndrome
- Prevention of Dental caries

What is happening now?

The report on child health surveillance (published under the title *Health for all Children*, Oxford Medical Publications) was approved by the British Paediatric Association, the British Medical Association, the Health Visitors Association and the Royal College of General Practitioners. The government health departments have also approved it. Child health surveillance is now mainly undertaken by general practitioners and health visitors with the community child health medical services providing a safety net service and secondary support.

A programme of child health surveillance has now been accepted by most Health Authorities in England and Wales. All doctors dealing with children should have a knowledge of what is involved in a child surveillance programme. The programme of the South Glamorgan Health Authority is given as an example (Table 12.1).

Table 12.1 South Glamorgan Health Authority Child Health Surveillance Programme, based on *Health for all Children*, Oxford Medical Publications

Test	Requirement for satisfactory coding	Examiner
Age 6 weeks (range 4–12 weeks)		
Weight and Head circumference (cm)		Doctor
Full physical examination	No significant abnormality	Doctor
Vision	Mother not concerned about eyesight, inspection normal including red reflex	Doctor
Hearing	Mother not concerned about hearing, baby not in high-risk category	Doctor
Hip check	Normal	
Testes	Descended	
Breast feeding	Fully breast fed up until the time of the examination	Doctor
Age 7–9 months		
Hearing test	Normal response to distraction test according to agreed criteria	Health visitor
Age 8 months (range 7–10 months)		
Weight		Doctor
Physical examination	No evidence of congenital heart disease	Doctor

Test	Requirement for satisfactory coding	Examiner
Vision	No concern about vision on the part of mother/examiner, no squint	Doctor
Hearing	No concern about hearing, no risk factors, check H/V distraction test	Doctor
Locomotion	Sits completely unsupported	Doctor
Hip check	Normal, i.e. abduction not limited and legs symmetrical with no maternal concern	Doctor
Testes	Descended	Doctor
Age 18 months		
Vision	No concern by mother/examiner, no squint	Health visitor
Hearing	No concern by mother, no risk factors	
Locomotion	Walks 5–6 steps completely independently	Health visitor
Speech/language	Understands simple instructions, points to named body parts, uses some understandable words	Health visitor
Behaviour	No concern by mother/examiner	Health visitor
Hip check	Normal, i.e. normal walking gait, symmetrical, abduction not limited	Health visitor
Age 3 years (range 33–42 months)		
Height	Measured and centiles recorded	Health visitor
Weight	Measured and centiles recorded	
Locomotion	Walks freely, including upright walking up and down stairs, gets to standing without rolling prone first	Health visitor
Vision	Inspection of eyes, observation of use and parental concern	Health visitor
Hearing	No concern/mother or examiner	Health visitor
Speech/language	Intellible speech/3 word combination	Health visitor

13 Physical problems

Congenital dislocation of the hip

Not all cases of congenital dislocation of the hip can be detected at birth. Therefore there should be surveillance of congenital dislocation of the hip (CDH) until the child is walking normally. Late diagnosis of CDH may lead to on-going problems with walking, multiple operations and later osteoarthritis. Early detection is highly worthwhile.

Risk factors for CDH include:

- Family history
- Female sex
- Breech presentation
- Cerebral palsy and other neurological diseases
- Other congenital malformations
- Asymmetry

If these conditions apply special care should be taken. If there is doubt the child should have an ultrasound examination of the hip and receive an expert orthopaedic opinion.

Detecting congenital dislocation of the hip in the child surveillance programme

In the first months of life CDH should be excluded by Barlow's and Ortolani's tests.

• Ortolani's Test: a test for dislocated hips. The child lies supine, the hips are flexed to a right angle and knees fully flexed. The femur is pushed firmly backwards and the gently abducted. If the hips is dislocated it slips into the acetabulum. This will be felt as a course clunk. This is different from the much finer click which is usually muscular.

• Barlow's Test: a test for dislocatable hips. The hip is abducted to 45°C and then tested to see if it is possible to push posteriorly and push the head in and out of the socket.

These tests should be used for the examination at 6 to 8 weeks. The child should also have had two examinations within 24 hours of birth and on discharge from the neonatal unit.

These tests are not suitable for older children, i.e. for the examination at 8 months and 18 months.

At the 8-month examination abduction should not be limited and the legs and creases should be symmetrical.

At 18 months there should be a normal walking gait which should be symmetrical and abduction should not be limited.

Referral of possible CDH is best done to an orthopaedic surgeon with a special interest in this problem.

Examination for undescended testes

Children at particular risk of undescended testes are:

• Those born pre-term
• Those born with low birth weight
• Those with an inguinal hernia

Examination should include palpation with the testis being gently manipulated along the path of descent. Often in true undescended testes the scrotum is underdeveloped on the side in question. In older boys retractile testes can be difficult to assess. A warm room and keeping handling to a minimum can help.

Examination is recommended at:

• 6 weeks, when testicular descent is noted

• 8 months when, if there is doubt, the child should be referred to a paediatric surgeon. If the testes are in the scrotum the parents should be told.

Congenital heart disease

Children should be examined for cardiovascular abnormalities at birth, 6 weeks and on one other occasion between 6 weeks and 5 years. An examination at 8 months if a doctor is going to be involved at that time is a particularly suitable time for this to take place. Referral of suspected cases should be to a paediatrician or paediatric cardiologist. The aim should now be to make a diagnosis if possible: reassure the parents if nothing is found and formulate a plan if abnormality is found. The use of echocardiography should mean that long periods of hospital follow-up for benign murmurs should not be needed.

Examination should include:

• Listening for murmurs. Remember that many murmurs heard in the first days of life are not significant and are probably due to late duct closure. Most cases of patent ductus arteriosus in the first years of life do not have a diastolic murmur. Refer urgently if there is cyanosis or the child is in heart failure. Benign murmurs are very common in the first years of life and are exacerbated by illness particularly febrile illness.

• Looking for cyanosis. Remember some cases of cyanotic heart disease, such as Fallot's tetrology, do not present at birth and the cyanosis develops slowly. Refer the neonate urgently if in doubt as duct closure may put the child's circulation suddenly in severe problems.

• Feeling for the femoral pulse. Remember that feeling these pulses may not be easy. If in doubt refer urgently as some cases of coarctation of the aorta deteriorate suddenly.

• Checking the child is not in failure. Remember that hepatomegaly may be the only physical sign of heart failure in infants. There may be a raised respiratory rate and shortness of breath on feeds. Refer urgently if in doubt.

In children with Down's syndrome an echocardiogram is now recommended because of the high instance of congenital heart disease, particularly AV canal defect.

Other common physical abnormalities that may be detected on the neonatal examination

Hydrocoeles

Hydrocoeles in the first weeks of life are common and resolve without treatment and the parents can be reassured. The only point of concern is that inguinal herniae are more common after hydrocoeles have resolved. Parents should be warned of this.

Inguinal herniae

Inguinal hernia should be referred to the paediatric surgeon because of the danger of strangulation. They are more common in pre-term babies and are unusual in girls where disorders of sexual differentiation should be excluded.

Umbilical hernia

Umbilical hernia is a common variation from normal which resolves without treatment. It is more common in Afro-Caribbean babies.

Hypospadias

Glandular hypospadias is as common as 1 in 50 male births. Usually it does not require treatment, although chordee may need attention. Further investigation (i.e. chromosomes) is not needed unless the testes are undescended. The parents should be reassured about future urinary and sexual function.

Penile hypospadias needs referral to the paediatric surgeon and full investigation.

Cleft lip and palate

Cleft lip with or without cleft palate is usually obvious and should be referred to a centre with plastic surgery and orthodontic input. Isolated cleft palate should be excluded with a finger in the mouth. This should also be referred urgently particularly because of the dangers of upper respiratory obstruction.

Single umbilical artery

Babies with a single umbilical artery without other congenital malformations do not, on the whole, need referral for further investigation.

Erupted teeth

Erupted teeth in the newborn usually do not cause problems apart from painful breast feeding. If they are loose they may need dental removal because of the danger of aspiration.

Stork marks

These naevi on the forehead and the nape of the neck fade with time and are not significant problems. Referral is not needed and parents should be reassured.

Strawberry naevus

These common raised lesions are not present at birth but appear in the first weeks of life. They get bigger to a maximum size between 6 months and a year. After that they fade gradually and are usually not visible after the age of 5 years. They are more common in pre-term babies. They do not need treatment. Referral is not needed and parents should be reassured.

Mongolian blue spot

These pigmented lesions with geographical edges are classically found on the back and sacrum. They fade over the first years of life. They are found most commonly in babies whose origins are from China, the Indian Subcontinent and Arab countries.

Hairy patch over the spine

Hairy patches over the spine may sometimes be of little significance, however, a significant proportion are associated with spinal dysraphism. There should be a low threshold for referral for investigation.

Anal dimple

Although pits over the spine are often associated with spinal dysraphism small pits near the anus do not have sinister significance and the parents can be reassured. Any question of discharge from a pit should be investigated.

Polydactyly

On the hands polydactyly can vary very much from whole extra fingers to small pieces of finger tissue attached by a thin band containing the blood supply. These are often tied off. However, this can sometimes leave painful remnants and if there is any doubt there should be referral to a paediatric or plastic surgeon. Polydactyly of the feet is usually less of a problem functionally for the child, however, if there is doubt referral is justified.

Talipes equinovarus

Talipes that does not correct should be referred urgently to the orthopaedic surgeon. Positional talipes which does correct can be treated with simple exercises at home and should not need referral.

14 Vision

Assessment of vision in the child surveillance programme

Vision should be informally assessed at all stages of the child surveillance programme. However, there are clear times in the programme where vision should be assessed (6–8 weeks, 8 months and 36–42 months). There are certain factors in the history which might mean that particular care should be taken with the assessment of the child's vision. These include:

- Family history of visual defects, such as cataracts etc.
- Concern during pregnancy (congenital rubella syndrome, toxoplasmosis etc.)
- Drugs during pregnancy
- Concern around birth, particularly birth trauma and pre-term
- Parents' concern regarding vision.
- Previous illness in a child, particularly meningitis, encephalitis etc.
- Injury to a child, particularly head injury

Visual problems that should be detected by the child surveillance programme

Visual problems that should be detected include:

- Cataract which may be inherited, linked to metabolic disease, due to congenital infections etc.
- Corneal opacities which may be due to metabolic disease, i.e. mucopolysaccharidoses, infections etc.
- Micro-ophthalmia
- Coloboma
- Infantile glaucoma (buphthalmos)
- Nystagmus which may be due to severe visual defect or congenital
- Albinism, a recessively inherited metabolic condition with nystagmus, visual defect and photophobia
- Retinopathy of prematurity, a proliferation of blood vessels and fibrous tissue due to oxygen sensitivity in pre-term babies. It may present as a mass behind the lens
- Retinoblastoma which may present as a white eye with a mass behind the lens. It needs urgent treatment and genetic counselling
- Toxocara infestation
- Severe refractive errors
- Retinal degenerations, in particular Leber's amaurosis, a disorder recessively inherited with severe visual defect
- Optic atrophy
- Congenital infections including rubella, toxoplasmosis, cytomegalovirus etc.
- Cortical blindness

Assessment of vision at various points in the child surveillance programme

Six to eight weeks

Major problems in vision should be able to be ascertained at this examination. The following should be enquired into:

- History from the mother. Is the baby beginning to look at her?
- Fixation. From 6 to 10 weeks a baby should be able to fixate on an object and failure to follow an object should result in referral for further assessment. This may be due to a visual problem or global delay.

• General examination of the eye, looking for micro-ophthalmia etc.
• Looking for lens opacities. The ophthalmoscope can be used to look for the 'red reflex' with any opacity being seen as a shadow obliterating either all or part of the reflex. Any suggestion of opacity should be referred to the ophthalmologist.
• Pupillary reactions.
• Squint. Any suggestion of a squint should be referred for further assessment by the ophthalmologists.
• Abnormal eye movements, i.e. nystagmus. Nystagmus may be an early sign of major visual problem.

Seven to ten months

• History from the mother. How does the baby use his or her vision?
• Visually directed reaction. The baby should see and pick up small objects. The baby should pick up a raisin with a finger–thumb grip by 10 months. He or she should have a sufficiently wide field of visual attention to be interested in small objects 3 m away.
• Squint. A squint is abnormal and should be referred.

Eighteen to twenty-four months

• History from the mother. How does the child use his or her vision? Are there any concerns?
• Check the child's vision around the room. He or she should be able to observe objects at a distance.
• Can the child pick up small objects?
• Squint. A squint is abnormal and should be referred.

Thirty-six to forty-two months

• History from the mother. Are there any concerns?
• Squint. A squint is abnormal and should be referred.
• The child should be able to recognize small objects and pictures with a field of vision of at least 3 m.

Tests involved in visual assessment

Squint

Remember that a broad bridge to the child's nose can give the impression of a squint without adequate testing the so called pseudo-squint. The two main types of squint that are seen in children are:

- The concomitant squint where the angle is the same in all directions of gaze and whichever eye is fixing. This is the commonest squint seen in children.
- The paralytic squint (incomitant squint) where the angle alters with different positions of gaze and with change of fixation of the eyes.

Tests used to screen for squint are:

- Corneal reflection test. A torch is shone into the eyes. In a normal child the reflections of the light are symmetrical in the pupils, if they are asymmetrical a squint should be suspected.
- The cover test. The child looks at a small object, each eye is covered in turn and in a normal child the eyes do not move. In a child with a squint there will be no movement when the squinting eye is covered, but when the normal eye is covered the squinting eye will move.

Testing for impaired visual acuity

The measurement of visual acuity presents difficulties in children under the age of 2.5 years. There are a number of tests that are available which include the STYCAR Tests (Sheridan Tests for young children and retardates) and the Sheridan Gardiner Tests. The Snellen Test Card provides the most satisfactory way of testing for visual problems and should be used as soon as practical.

Tests for visual acuity can be divided into minimum observable, minimum separable and qualitative tests:

Minimum observable tests

These are tests that establish the smallest object visible to the child. They include:

- Picking up small objects or sweets (from 8 months onwards) such as hundreds and thousands, cake decoration balls, raisins or smarties assessing near vision in small children.
- STYCAR graded ball test in which small balls are rolled 3 m from the child. The smallest is 3 mm in diameter.

Minimum separable tests

These are tests that measure the ability to separate visual stimulae. They include:

- STYCAR miniature toy tests in which the child is required to distinguish between a toy knife, fork and spoon at 3 m.
- Letter matching tests in which a child matches single letters with those held by a parent. This may be at 3 m (STYCAR) or at 6 m (Sheridan Gardiner). For children aged 3.5 to 4.5 years use five letters and for children aged 4.5 to 5.5 years use seven letters.
- Shape recognition tests.
- The Snellen test which involves full lines of letters and should be used as soon as practical. It is the test that is usually involved with screening for visual defects at school age.

Qualitative tests

Qualitative tests observe visual function such as person or object recognition and response to television. They do not formally assess visual acuity but give a useful guide to function.

Defects in colour vision

Defects in colour vision usually involve red–green discrimination. There are three main conditions:

- Protanopia: a deficiency of appreciation of red. Protan colour blindness.
- Deuteranopia: a deficiency of green vision with confusion of colours. Deutan colour blindness.
- Tritanopia: sensitivity to blue is impaired. This is very rare.

Protan and deutan colour blindness are inherited as sex-linked recessive conditions and therefore are much more common in boys than girls. They are due to separate genes. Tritan colour blindness is inherited as an autosomal dominant condition with limited penetrance.

The Ishihara test plates (H.K. Lewis and Co., London) are most commonly used as an efficient screening test for red–green defects. Numbers are seen on the plates by those people with normal vision and not by those with red–green defects. Some tracing paths are included for young children. The Ishihara test unfortunately does not distinguish very well between those colour defects which are of practical importance and those which are not. It is therefore best used as a screening test, with the second edition of the City University test (Keeler UK Series, London) being used for those that 'fail' it. In this test ten plates provide a display of five coloured spots. There are a number of other tests for colour vision which are sometimes used.

A flow chart for use in schools for testing 12-year-old boys would be:

Ishihara test – if failed, repeat.
If failed, try the City University test.
If failed, write a letter to the parents with employment advice.

There are a number of jobs and careers which need perfect colour vision. These include the armed forces, electrical work, work in civil aviation, navigation at sea and on the railways.

15 Hearing

Detecting hearing loss in the child surveillance programme

Children with particular points on the history or examination need special attention for hearing in the child surveillance programme. If special attention is given to these points, in particular parental concern, many cases of hearing loss can be detected before a child is old enough for distraction tests at 7–9 months. Indeed, many centres are now testing these children as babies by electrophysiological testing such as *p*rogrammable *o*toacoustic *em*ission by *s*timulation (POEMS). These points include:

- Birth weight less 1500 g.
- Family history of childhood hearing impairment
- Congenital infections (congenital rubella, toxoplasmosis, cytomegalovirus)
- Congenital malformations including craniofacial abnormalities (such as cleft palate) and first arch abnormalities (such as the Treacher Collins syndrome etc.)
- Severe hyperbilirubinaemia during the neonatal period
- Severe birth asphyxia
- Persistent otitis media, particularly chronic secretory otitis media
- Meningitis, particularly *Haemophilus influenzae* and encephalitis

- Head injuries
- Drugs such as aminoglycosides

Parental concern on hearing

Parental concern can be formulated by a hearing check list such as developed in Nottingham for parents.

Hints for Parents ————————————————————

"Can your baby hear you?"

Here is a checklist of some of the general signs you can look for
in your baby's first year:—

YES/NO

Shortly after birth
Your baby should be startled by a sudden loud noise such as hand clap or
a door slamming and should blink or open his eyes widely to such sounds.

By 1 Month
Your baby should be beginning to notice sudden prolonged sounds like the
noise of a vacuum cleaner and he should pause and listen to them when
they begin.

By 4 Months
He should quieten or smile to the sound of your voice even when he cannot
see you. He may also turn his head or eyes toward you if you come up from
behind and speak to him from the side.

By 7 Months
He should turn immediately to your voice across the room to very quiet
noises made on each side if he is not too occupied with other things.

By 9 Months
He should listen attentively to familiar everyday sounds and search for very
quiet sounds made out of sight. He should also show pleasure in babbling
loudly and tunefully.

By 12 Months
He should show some response to his own name and to other familiar
words. He may also respond when you say 'no' and 'bye bye' even when he
cannot see any accompanying gesture.

> Your health visitor will perform a routine hearing screening test on your
> baby between six and eight months of age. She will be able to help and
> advise you at any time before or after this test if you are concerned
> about your baby and his development. If you suspect that your baby is
> not hearing normally, either because you cannot answer yes to the items
> above or for some other reason, then seek advice from your health
> visitor.

©
Produced by Dr. Barry McCormick
Children's Hearing Assessment Centre, General Hospital, Nottingham NG1 6HA
Printed by The Sherwood Press (Nottingham) Limited

Detecting hearing loss in specific parts of the child surveillance programme

Six to eight weeks

- Enquire into points of concern, i.e. birth and family history
- Introduce a hearing check list (if not done by the health visitor) and enquire about parental concern regarding hearing
- Check startle response to a loud sound. This may be very difficult to interpret

Seven to nine months

All children should have a distraction hearing test between 7 and 9 months. This test is based on the child's ability to localize sound. At this age a child should be able to turn his or her head directly to a noise from behind. Later children may lose interest because of an increasing distractibility and tests become unreliable and difficult.

For a distraction test to take place two trained people are essential: a distractor and a tester. The tester should be behind and to one side of the child. The sound level of the room should be quiet.

The distractor takes the child's attention and stimulates the child with toys etc. This stimulation is then withdrawn and a testing sound is put to one side of the child. Care must be taken not to be within the child's visual field, which extends beyond 180°. Both sides should be tested. The stimulus should be presented:

- At a distance of 1 m from the ear
- At the same height as the child's ear
- Behind the lateral angle of vision

The stimuli used are frequency specific:

- High-frequency stimuli such as an 'SS' sound or a Nuffield or Manchester rattle and a portable Freefield audiometer in distraction testing and 4 kHz warble tones

- Low-frequency stimuli such as warble tones at 500 Hz, a hum (such as a nursery rhyme), a low quiet voice, i.e. 'oo-oo' or 'mm-mm', or a minimal voiced sentence (excluding sibilants)

If there is any doubt, the test should be repeated in a month's time and if there is still doubt a referral should be made for a clear audiological assessment.

Examination at eighteen to twenty-four months

Hearing may be difficult to assess as children are too easily distracted by other things for a distraction test and may be too young for cooperative tests.

- Refer if in doubt
- Assess history, parental concern
- Children should be babbling at 10 months and have single words at 21 months

Thirty-six to forty-two months

- At this time examination is essentially an assessment of communication and language.
- All speech-delayed children should have an audiological assessment.

Hearing tests used in referrals from child surveillance programmes

Hearing tests measure the response to sounds:

- Intensity is measured in decibels (db): 20–30 db is a whisper, 60 db conversational voice, 110 db a shout and 140 db pain.
- Frequency of a sound wave is measured in cycles per second or hertz (Hz). The important speech range is from 250 Hz to 4000 Hz (4 kHz). The human ear should be able to receive frequencies between 20 Hz and 20 000 Hz (20 kHz).

Speech is a mixture of low-frequency and high-frequency sounds. Defects may only be recognized when impaired speech comprehension is present.

Hearing tests in pre-school children

Children over the age of 3 or 4 years can be tested by pure tone audiology with headphones and pure tones. Before the age of 3 or 4 years other hearing testing methods have to be used.

Tests for babies

Babies who are thought to be at specific risk of hearing loss can be screened for hearing loss. Methods used include *p*rogrammable *o*toacoustic *e*mission by *s*timulation (POEMS), brain stem evoked response audiometry (BSER). Another method is the auditory response cradle.

Distraction tests

See above.

Speech tests

Speech tests can be useful for testing young children who are not able to use pure tone audiometry. The child sits with the mother in front of the tester. The child can be shown special chosen objects (Kendal Toy Tests or the McCormick Toy Test). The child is told the name of each item and then asked to 'show me' the item concerned. The tester must ensure the child is unable to lip read.

Performance and cooperative tests

In these tests the child is asked to make a specific response each time he or she hears a sound. The simplest approach is to find the quietest level at which the child can distinguish between simple familiar instructions or requests.

Children with a mental age over 2.5 years should be capable of undertaking a simple pre-audiometry conditioning procedure known as a performance test, i.e. the child places a toy in a container each time a sound is heard. This is usually done together with a freefield audiometer.

Electrical response audiometry

In some cases, particularly in children with evidence of delayed development and speech delay, there can be serious doubt about whether the children can hear or not. This question is unable to be answered by standard distraction or conditioning tests. In this case electrical responses are noted in the pathways to the brain stem and cortex after a sound. There are two main tests that are used:

- Electrocochleography (ECOG) which needs a general anaesthetic. A needle with an electrode is inserted through the tympanic membrane and rests on the promontory in the middle ear and action potentials produced by the cochlea are recorded.
- Brain stem evoked responses (BSER) which are recorded from electrodes on the surface, usually on the scalp, mastoid and forehead. The transmission of the auditory signal from the cochlea to the cortex is recorded on the EEG, usually by computer analysis.

Impedance

Impedance is measured using a tympanometer. It is a useful technique to be used together with audiological assessment. It gives an assessment of the mobility of the tympanic membranes. It can be useful in diagnosing middle ear disease. A probe is inserted into the external ear canal which has a sound source and a microphone to measure reflected sound energy.

Pure tone audiometry

The pure tone audiometry technique requires headphones and an audiometer generating pure tones. Children 4 years old and over can usually tolerate the headphones and respond to the sound. Air and bone conduction are measured and the response shown on an audiogram. Cross-conduction of sounds can be a problem in unilateral hearing loss. 'Masking' the non-tested ear with other sound is used to overcome this problem.

Screening for hearing loss in the school programme

All children entering schools should have their hearing screened by pure tone audiometry.

Each ear is separately tested. Four frequencies are usually tested (500 Hz, 1, 2, 4 kHz) at a fixed sound level (usually 25 db).

Managing the deaf child

Like all handicaps it is essential that a multidisciplinary approach is undertaken with deaf children. A number of different professionals need to be involved. These include:

- Teachers for the deaf
- Audiologists
- Paediatricians with an expertise in audiology
- Speech therapists

Hearing aids

Hearing aids amplify sounds for the deaf child. They are an important part of the management of a deaf child. The selection of a suitable hearing aid needs to be made by a paediatric audiologist in consultation with the teachers for the hearing impaired.

Aids have a mould that fits in the ear. The fitting of this mould is important and will need altering as the child grows. Aids can be:

- Behind the ear
- In the ear
- A body worn aid
- Bone conducting aids

Methods of education used with deaf children

Hearing impaired children can either attend:

● Normal schools
● Normal schools with special facilities for the hearing impaired
● Special schools for the hearing impaired

Which type of school is chosen depends on the child, the family and local conditions. Many deaf children lip read but many teachers for the hearing impaired believe that they should have sign language as well. This can be:

● British sign language
● Signed English
● Finger spelling
● Makaton (particularly useful for the child with learning difficulties as well as deafness)

16 Development

In the past a number of screening tests were used to detect problems of development in children. The child surveillance programme aims to detect problems in development whose recognition should be easily achievable such as delayed walking. These developmental milestones were chosen by the Working Party on Child Surveillance to be those, on the best evidence available, that were worthwhile detecting.

Assessment of development at various points in the child surveillance programme

Six to eight weeks

Only a limited assessment of development is possible at 6–8 weeks. What is possible in the general examination includes:

- Babies should be smiling by 6 weeks. Allow for the baby being pre-term.
- Babies should be noting tone when bringing them from the supine to sitting position.
- Moro reflex and spontaneous limb movements which should be symmetrical.

Seven to ten months

A definite criterion is:

• Locomotion. Babies should sit completely unsupported. Babies should be sitting by 10 months. Most babies are sitting by 8 months.

Other points that may be noticed during the examination include:

• No head lag when pulled to sitting.
• The baby beginning to babble.
• The baby beginning to understand its environment. It may point at an object.
• By 10 months a baby should pick up a small object (i.e. a raisin) with a finger–thumb grip. Before this it may rake the object.
• Crawling is a very variable and unreliable milestone.

Eighteen to twenty-four months

Definite criteria include:

• Locomotion. A child should be able to walk five or six steps completely independently.
• Speech/language. A child should understand simple instructions, point to named body parts and use some understandable words.

Other points that may be noticed during the examination include:

• Children at this age can usually name objects and pictures (i.e. common household objects and large toys). There is a wide variation in the use of spoken language at this age.
• The beginnings of imaginative play.
• A child should be able to fetch a named object.

Thirty-six to forty-two months

Definite criteria include:

• Locomotion. A child should be able to walk freely, including upright, walking up and down stairs and get to a standing position without rolling prone first.

- Speech. Clearly intelligible speech should be heard, although it may have some unclear syllables.

Other points that may be noticed during the examination include:

- Recognition of parts of the body, pictures etc.
- Many children will recognize big and little, under and on.
- Children will play meaningfully with toys and with adults.

Problems in development

These can be divided into those of:

- Motor development
- Speech and language delay
- Global delay

Delay in motor development

Normal patterns of motor development

There may be wide normal variations in motor development, particularly in the age of walking. There are familial factors that should be taken into account. Crawling is a very variable milestone and of little value as a tool in developmental assessment. Some normal children bottom shuffle which may be associated with physiological delayed walking. This is usually inherited as a dominant gene.

Milestones in motor development

- No head lag when pulled to sitting. Mean age: 3.5 months (90th centile 5 months).
- Rolls over prone–supine. Mean age: 4.5 months (90th centile 7.5 months).
- Safe sitting at least 5 seconds. Mean age: 6.5 months (90th centile 8 months).

- Getting to sitting from lying. Mean age: 9 months (90th centile 11.5 months).
- Getting to standing. Mean age: 9 months (90th centile 12.5 months).
- Walking five steps. Mean age: 13.5 months (90th centile 17 months).
- Walk up steps independently. Mean age: 16.5 months (90th centile 21.5 months).
- Pedalling a tricycle. Mean age: 30 months (90th centile 42 months).
- Balancing on one foot. Mean age: 30 months (90th centile 42 months).

Based on Bryant, G.M., Davis, K.J., Newcombe, R., *Developmental Medicine and Child Neurology*, 1979, **21**, 353–64.

Causes of motor delay

Normal variation

There is normal variation especially if there is a family history or bottom shuffling.

Neglect

Many deprived children have delayed motor and other milestones.

Chronic illness

Any severe illness such as cyanotic heart disease or chronic renal failure will retard motor milestones.

Congenital dislocation of the hip

This causes motor delay if not diagnosed in first weeks of life.

Spinal dysraphism

Exclude spinal dysraphism by examination for hairy patch on the spine and spinal X-ray.

Cerebral palsy

Note birth history but remember that not all children with cerebral palsy have had perinatal problems. Cerebral palsy children can be globally delayed or have delay just in the motor milestones.

Duchenne muscular dystrophy

Many Duchenne boys present with delayed walking. About 60% of them also have speech delay. Exclude by serum creatine phosphate kinase (CPK) which is grossly raised, i.e. several thousand IU.

Congenital myopathies

These present as a floppy infant. Diagnosis can be made by muscle biopsy.

Spinal muscular atrophy (SMA)

This presents again as a floppy infant. It can either be fatal in the first months of life (Werdnig–Hoffman Disease) or the infant can survive into childhood (intermediate SMA).

Joint laxity

May present with motor delay.

Speech and language delay

Normal patterns of communication

There are wide variations in the patterns of the development of speech and communication. It is useful to take a family history of late speaking as delay in language development may be inherited. Milestones that are valuable in assessment include:

- Localization of sound. Mean age 4 months (90th centile 7 months).

- Understanding words for familiar objects. Mean age: 18 months (90th centile 22 months).
- Meaningful two-word combinations. Mean age: 18 months (90th centile 24 months).
- Naming pictures. Mean age: 20 months (90th centile 24 months).
- Intelligible speech. Mean age 30 months (90th centile 42 months).

(Based on Bryant *et al.*, *ibid.*)

Development of individual sounds

As speech develops some syllables are unclear and there may be 'infantile substitutions', i.e. 't' and 'd' being used for 'k' and 'g'. For instance:

- At 3 years children should be able to say vowels and m,n,p,b.
- At 4 years children should be able to say t,d,k,g.

Causes of speech delay

If comprehension of the spoken word is impaired and there is delay in other areas consider:

- Neglect
- Global delay

If comprehension of the spoken word is impaired and there is no delay in other areas consider:

- Deafness if the child does not hear.
- Autism if the child hears, but does not communicate by other means.
- Receptive language disorders if the child hears and uses alternative methods of communication.

If comprehension of the spoken word is normal for age and there is delay in other areas consider:

- Immaturity, neglect or expressive language disorder if the child has limited language, but clear speech.

• Dysarthria if the child has plentiful language which is not intelligible with consistent errors, particularly if there is a physical diagnosis such as cerebral palsy that might explain this problem.
• Dyspraxia if the child has plentiful language which is not intelligible with inconsistent errors.

General assessment of the child with speech and language delay

The assessment of a child with speech delay should include:

• A full family history
• A full pregnancy and birth history
• An expert medical examination to exclude particular syndromes
• An audiological assessment
• A full developmental assessment such as a Griffith's test
• Special tests including chromosomes, creatine phosphate kinase (CPK) in a boy to exclude Duchenne muscular dystrophy which may present as speech delay, TORCH (Toxoplasmosis – Rubella – Cytomegalovirus-Herpes) screen.
• Speech therapy assessment

Global delayed development

Children with globally delayed development on assessment may be divided into those who will go on to have learning difficulties and those who have delayed milestones which are due to:

• Neglect. Delayed development in deprived situations may take months or even years to revert to normal when the child is placed in a loving home.
• Chronic illness.
• Normal variation.

Children with learning difficulties (used to be called mental retardation or handicap) are usually divided into:

• Severe with an IQ less than 50
• Mild to moderate with an IQ above 50

Causes of global learning difficulties

The majority of children with learning difficulties do not have a recognized cause. However, as the diagnosis of genetic disorders gets better more and more causes of this problem are being recognized.

There is rarely any treatment for children with learning difficulties. Nevertheless, it is valuable to make an exact diagnosis in these children because:

* It gives a prognosis
* It enables exact genetic counselling to be done
* It prevents uncertainty for the parents

Remember, if development is regressing think of a degenerative disorder. Causes of children with global delay include:

* Chromosome disorders. Down's syndrome and *Cri du Chat* syndrome are well defined. The Fragile X syndrome is also an important cause of delay in boys. There are many other less common chromosomal abnormalities as well and all children with global delay should have their chromosomes checked.
* Dysmorphic syndromes. There are a large number of dysmorphic syndromes associated with global delay. Dysmorphic features should be looked for on examination.
* Well-recognized diseases. Tuberose sclerosis, neurofibromatosis, Duchenne dystrophy etc. may all be associated with global delay.
* Structural developmental problems of the CNS such as microcephaly.
* Infection during pregnancy, e.g. TORCH (Toxoplasmosis–Rubella–Cytomegalovirus–Herpes) infections.
* Biochemical disorders. Phenylketonuria should be now eliminated by neonatal screening. Others are individually rare.
* Birth asphyxia and other perinatal problems. Some cases of cerebral palsy are globally delayed.
* Hypothyroidism should be eliminated by the neonatal screening process.
* Severe illness in the first year of life. This includes meningitis, encephalitis, infantile spasms etc.
* Trauma to the brain.

Investigation

All globally delayed children should have:

- A full history taken including pregnancy, birth and family history
- A full clinical examination including looking for dysmorphic features
- Chromosomes investigated
- A TORCH screen
- Creatine phosphate kinase (CPK) test in boys

Many should have:

- A mucopolysaccharide screen
- A thyroid screen
- Urinary aminoacids tested
- Radiological investigation for CNS malformations.

Tests used to assess development

- Denver Developmental Screening Test. This is a test developed in the USA and modified by Bryant for British children. (Available from Test Agency, High Wycombe, Bucks.)
- Griffith's Test (Test Agency). The standard test in the UK for detailed assessment of a child's development after problems have been raised in child surveillance. It is divided into the following sections:

  Locomotor
  Personal/social
  Hearing and speech
  Eye and hand coordination
  Performance
  Practical reasoning

- Schedule of growing skills (Bellman and Cash) based on the Mary Sheridan Tests.
- Speech therapy tests commonly used by speech therapists such as Reynell Developmental Language Scales or

Edinburgh Articulation Tests (E. and F. Livingstone, Edin-burgh). Metaphon and PACS (Nelson, Windsor, Berks) give a useful profile for intervention.

Patterns of malformation with children with global delay

Chromosome abnormalities

- Down's syndrome

  Hypotonia
  Flat faces
  Small ears
  Slanted palpebral fissures
  Speckling of Iris (Brushfield's spots)
  Short metacarpals and phalanges
  Single palmer creases
  Wide gap between 2nd and 3rd toes

- Trisomy 13

  Central cleft lip
  Polydactyly
  Microcephaly with sloping forehead
  Scalp defects

- Trisomy 18

  Clenched hand
  Prominent occiput
  Hypertonicity
  Feet with prominent curved heels – 'rocker-bottom' feet

- *Cri du Chat* syndrome (5p- syndrome)

  Cat-like cry as a baby
  Microcephaly
  Downward slant of the palpebral fissures

NB There are a number of relatively rare chromosome abnormality syndromes associated with learning difficulties and chromosomes should be checked on all such children.

Other syndromes

- Angelman syndrome (Happy puppet syndrome)
  Jerky gait ('puppet'-like)
  Paroxysms of laughter
  Characteristic facies

- Ataxia–Telangiectasia syndrome
  Ataxia
  Telangiectasia
  Lymphopenia
  Immune deficit

- Borjeson–Forssman–Lehmann syndrome
  Large ears
  Hypogonadism

- Cockayne syndrome
  Changes similar to senility but beginning in infancy
  Retinal degeneration
  Photosensitivity of thin skin

- Coffin–Siris syndrome
  Hypoplastic to absent fifth finger and toenails
  Coarse facies

- Cornelia de Lange syndrome
  Short stature prenatal onset
  Bushy eyebrows
  Eyebrows meeting in the middle (Synophrys)

- Dubowitz syndrome
  Peculiar facies
  Infantile eczema
  Small stature
  Mild microcephaly

- Fragile X syndrome
  Mild connective tissue dysplasia
  Macro-orchidism (large testes)
  Prominent jaw

- Hurler syndrome (Mucopolysaccharidosis I)

  Coarse facies
  Stiff joints
  Cloudy cornea

- Hunter syndrome (Mucopolysaccharidosis II)

  Coarse facies
  Growth deficiency
  Stiff joints

- Menkes 'Kinky Hair' syndrome

  Progressive deterioration with seizures
  Twisted and fractured hair

- Miller–Dieker syndrome (Lissencephaly)

  Microcephaly with ridging and furrowing in central forehead

- Neurofibromatosis

  See text

- Phenyketonuria – fetal effects from maternal disease

- Phenytoin–foetal phenytoin syndrome

- Prader–Willi syndrome

  Hypotonia
  Obesity
  Small hands and feet

- Rubella–congenital rubella syndrome

  Nerve deafness
  Retinopathy
  Cataracts
  Failure to thrive

- Rubinstein–Taybi syndrome

  Broad thumbs and toes
  Slanted palpebral fissures
  Hypoplastic maxilla

- Sanfilippo syndrome (Mucopolysaccharidosis III)

Mild coarse facies
Mild stiff joints
Mental deficiency

- Seckel syndrome (Seckel's bird-headed dwarf)

  Severe short stature
  Microcephaly
  Prominent nose

- Sjögren–Larsson syndrome

  Ichthyosis
  Spasticity

- Smith–Lemli–Opitz syndrome

  Moderate short stature
  Anteverted nostrils
  Ptosis of eyelids
  Hypospadias
  Cryptorchidism

- Sotos syndrome (cerebral gigantism)

  Large size
  Large hands and feet
  Poor coordination

- Sturge–Weber syndrome

  Flat facial hemangiomata
  Meningeal hemangiomata with seizures

- Tuberose sclerosis

  See text

- Williams syndrome

  Prenatal growth deficiency
  Mild to moderate learning difficulties
  Aortic stenosis or pulmonary stenosis
  Blue eyes
  Depressed nasal bridge

17 Behavioural problems

Many parents perceive that their children have behavioural problems. Many of these children have a variant of normal behaviour. Children in their toddler years normally display negativism: they may refuse to sleep, feed or toilet train to search for their independence.

Children in the first five years of life must learn to interact with other children. This process is helped by going to playgroup and nursery. Arranging playgroup and nursery places for children is an important part of the modern management of the under fives. The doctor caring for children can influence the provision of playgroup places for children.

Children need:

- A loving environment
- Adequate play opportunities at home
- A reasonably structured life
- A regular routine

If they lack these, significant behavioural problems may result. Although most perceived behavioural problems in children are variations from normal, severe behavioural problems may be signs of:

- Emotional abuse
- Developmental delay

Dealing with behavioural problems

Most behavioural problems can be dealt with by simple advice in a primary care setting. Referral should only be rarely needed and in most cases should be to either:

- A child psychologist
- A paediatrician (especially when there are accompanying physical problems or abuse is suspected)
- A child psychiatrist

General assessment

All children with behavioural problems should have a full assessment:

- The frequency of the problem and precipitating factors should be ascertained. A chart may be useful in assessing this.
- A full social history needs to be taken. The child should be seen as part of the family as a whole. Marriage problems, job problems within the family and family illness may well disrupt the normal routine of a child and exacerbate difficulties with behaviour. Parents with young children may often have very limited opportunities to go out together and may get very limited support from relatives.
- Medical factors must be considered, e.g. drugs, food allergy. This is rare but often parents perceive it as a major cause, particularly an allergy or intolerance to food dyes.
- Check for developmental delay. Developmental delay may precipitate behavioural problems in children, particularly when they get frustrated with their lack of ability.

General treatment

- Any obvious factors in the medical and social history should be dealt with if possible.
- Time off for the mother and child should be arranged with periods of alternative care. Attendance at playgroup or nursery should be encouraged.

- Good behaviour should be supported, bad behaviour not encouraged or rewarded. A chart with stars for good behaviour and rewards for so many stars is often helpful.
- A routine for the child needs to be established.
- A plan of action should be agreed with the parents for monitoring the results.
- A gradual withdrawal from a particular pattern of behaviour is more likely to be effective than a sudden one.
- Smacking is rarely effective and paradoxically may make things worse as it often brings the rewards to the child of attention and the parent feeling guilty.

Particular behavioural problems

Sleep problems

There are three types of sleeping difficulty:

- Difficulty in settling at bed time
- Waking throughout the night
- Settling and waking difficulties together

Many children normally spend parts of the nights with their parents and this should really not be viewed as outside of normal development. It may of course be very trying to parents.

Settling difficulties need the establishment of a set bed time routine with stories etc. They may be helped by making sure:

- The child is not hungry. It may be worth giving supper before going to bed such as a bowl of cereal
- The child is not too hot or too cold
- A warm bath is part of the routine
- The child has not outgrown the cot

Waking difficulties respond to a gradual withdrawal of the parent's intervention in a 'behavioural way'. The habit of drinking frequently throughout the day and night can exacerbate the problem.

Temper tantrums

Temper tantrums can be disabling for both the child and parents. They tend to resolve by the age of 5 years. Treatment requires:

- Temper tantrums should never be rewarded
- Rewards for good behaviour associated with a star chart
- Dealing with associated problems
- The tantrums themselves can be helped in young children by sending the child to a part of the room designated as a naughty corner or naughty chair. Holding the child on the lap in a firm but loving way until the tantrum is over is also an effective way of handling the situation.

Hyperactivity

- Many children in their toddler years can be very active normally and hyperactivity should not be regarded as a disease.
- Active children need a structured day with structured play opportunities. They respond to playgroup and nursery well.
- Are food dyes significant? There is no evidence that food dyes of the tartrazine type do children any good and it is wise to avoid these in all children if possible. A few children may be intolerant to these dyes. This can be demonstrated by a test dose (prepared by the pharmacy). Food dyes are not a major cause of 'hyperactivity' in children however.

Breath holding attacks

- Breath holding attacks where a child holds his or her breath after either being thwarted or being hurt can be very frightening to the parents and to the child. Eventually the child breathes again when the respiratory centre takes over.
- Further investigation is seldom needed as the history should exclude fits.
- The child should be reassured and cuddled during the attack, NOT turned upside down, given artificial respiration, slapped on the back etc.
- The parents should be reassured that children do not come to harm during these attacks.

Eating difficulties

Many under fives may refuse to eat for their parents which causes great anxiety. It is usually part of normal negativism. An assessment should include:

- Monitoring growth. The vast majority of children presenting with this problem are growing normally and the parents should be reassured.
- Monitoring diet. Some children have much of their calories as milk and this should be gradually changed. The child should sit with the family at regular meals. Snacks should be discouraged.

Parents should:

- Never force feed. Advise that the child should think it is a matter of indifference to the parents whether the child eats or not.
- Be given reassurance.

18 Helping the child with special needs

Any approach to a child with special needs should be both:

- Problem orientated
- Multidisciplinary

The multidisciplinary team should include:

- The parents
- Doctors – the paediatrician, general practitioner and specialized doctors such as orthopaedic and plastic surgeons
- Therapists – physiotherapists, occupational therapists and speech therapists
- Teachers – who may be specialists in the hearing or vision impaired or in special education
- Psychologists – who may be clinical or educational
- Health visitors and other nurses involved with children
- Social workers
- Orthotists and bioengineers
- Nursery nurses and play therapists

Such a multidisciplinary team will need to look at the problems the child has and will need to formulate a problem list and plan. Such a plan will include:

- Making a diagnosis
- Confirming the prognosis
- Making sure genetic issues are considered
- Deciding what adaptions might be necessary in the home to deal with the child's handicap

- Deciding what education the child should receive together with the Education Authority
- Deciding what therapy is going to be needed
- Dealing with associated problems of hearing and vision
- Deciding what mobility aids are needed and whether a wheelchair is going to be needed, if so what type
- Deciding whether any other special aids are needed
- Deciding whether respite or alternative care are needed
- Ensuring the family is receiving the benefits they are entitled to

Mobility for the child with special needs

Mobility is vital for the child with special needs. If a child can either walk, ambulate with help or use a wheelchair morale is improved and independent living is possible. Mobility can be helped by:

- Walking aids. These are particularly of value in cerebral palsy. They can be used in front of the child or at the back of the child (Kaye Walker).
- Hand walking aids
- Long leg callipers
- Swivel walkers. These are a low energy aid to ambulation. The child makes a side-to-side movement and as the centre of gravity is in the front the child moves forward. They were developed for paraplegics but can be used in situations where muscle power is reduced such as Duchenne muscular dystrophy and cerebral palsy.
- Hip guidance orthoses. These orthotic aids are used in children with spina bifida
- Wheelchairs

Wheelchairs

Wheelchairs are at present provided by the regional Artificial Limb and Appliance Centres (ALACs). In the future this role may be taken over by District Health Authorities. The ALACs have specialized technicians working with them, however, the advice of an occupational therapist is vital in the assessment of the use of a wheelchair. Outside electric wheelchairs are not at present provided by the ALACs and have to be provided by charity.

When considering a wheelchair ask:

- Who will operate it?
- Will the chair be used outside?
- Is the child restless and needing restraint?
- Does the child need postural support?
- Should the chair be able to fold?
- Who will maintain the wheelchair?
- Where will the chair be stored and who will service it?

Wheelchairs may need a number of modifications and adjustments if they are going to be comfortable and useful for the child. These include assessing and adjusting:

- The angle of the back
- The position of the headrest
- The position of the foot support
- The need for restraint
- The type of side support
- The number and type of cushions
- The indications for specially positioned shoes
- The need to inhibit regression of deformity
- The need to fit other appliances such as short leg callipers

Adapting the home for a child with special needs

Adaptions to the home are vital for the child with special needs. The occupational therapist has the major role in giving advice to the family. In most circumstances the Social Services Department is responsible for the adaptions that are needed within the home. They normally have their own occupational therapist who should liaise with the multidisciplinary team.

Although the Social Services Department of the County

Council, London or Metropolitan Borough (or in the case of council housing the District Council) has a special responsibility under the law to provide such adaptions that are necessary there are often delays. It is therefore a good idea to plan for any adaptions that are needed as soon as possible.

Sometimes adaptions to a particular house are impractical and the best advice that can be given is for the family to buy or rent a new house.

Adaptions may be to:

● Improve access to the home by providing outside ramps, increasing door widths etc.
● Improve access within the home by providing internal ramps, stair lifts, internal lifts etc. Sometimes it is better to build or adapt downstairs rooms as bedrooms and bathrooms rather than provide lifts for the wheelchair.
● Provide hoists, wheelchair accessible showers for toileting and bathing.

Dealing with common individual problems

Autism

Autism is a difficult and distressing condition that is best regarded as a severe communication disorder. About 75% of these children have severe learning difficulties. Autism does not have one cause but seems to be a behaviour disorder that has a number of causes.

Rutter has outlined the four essential features of autism:

● Delayed and deviant language development which has certain defined features and is out of keeping with the child's intellectual level.
● Impaired social development which has a number of special characteristics and is out of keeping with the child's intellectual level.
● Insistence on sameness as shown by stereotyped play patterns, abnormal preoccupations or resistance to change.
● Onset before the age of 30 months.

The speech delay may be severe. These children's behaviour

may involve rituals, obsessions and stereotypes. The management of these children is very difficult and the prognosis not good. They need a combination of specialized educational, psychological and speech therapy input. The load on the family is severe and residential schooling may be needed.

Asperger's syndrome

This name is given to children who have a behavioural syndrome not unlike autism but less severe with early language development not being delayed. The behaviour is solitary and obsessive. The personality is often difficult. Like autism a combined educational and psychological approach may be useful.

Cerebral palsy

Children with cerebral palsy have a large range of problems from minimal disability to severe physical handicap with severe global delay. The children may be of normal intelligence or have learning difficulties. Cerebral palsy is a non-progressive condition.

Cerebral palsy can be considered in the following ways.

Hemiplegia

In the first months asymmetry of hand movements and fisting may be noted. By the age of 1 year there should be increased tone and reflexes on the affected side. Sitting and crawling are usually delayed. Some of these children are bottom shufflers and have delayed walking. Hemiplegias can be congenital or acquired, either in the neonatal period or in the years following this.

Spastic cerebral palsy

In these conditions there is bilateral brain damage, feeding may be delayed and there are delayed motor milestones. Spastic cerebral palsy can be divided into:

- Spastic diplegia. This may be associated with perinatal

problems. The main signs are in the lower limbs. In order to walk there are excessive compensatory movements in the upper half of the body.

● Severe quadriplegia. This is usually associated with microcephaly and is often associated with birth asphyxia and post-natal brain injury.

The diagnosis of spastic cerebral palsy may be difficult in the first months as tone is variable:

● Some patients have marked spasticity in the first months of life
● Some are hypotonic

There may be microcephaly and head circumference needs to be monitored.

Signs later on include:

● Delays in motor development, particularly parachute reactions
● Persistent abnormal patterns such as the asymmetrical tonic neck reflex where the head is turned and the arm extended and symmetrical tonic reflex where the neck is extended, the arms extend and the knees flex
● Brisk tendon reflexes with clonus

Athetoid cerebral palsy

This again may be related to perinatal problems, usually associated with spasticity. The athetoid movements appear from 1 to 3 years. The child may be normal mentally. The prognosis for these children is often better than for children with spastic diplegia and walking may be achieved in late childhood. It may often be associated with dysarthria.

Minimal cerebral palsy

There are some clumsy children who have mild, but definite physical signs which may be described as having minimal cerebral palsy.

Ataxic cerebral palsy

This term is best reserved for children with definite cerebellar signs, associated with global delay.

Associated problems

Children with cerebral palsy may have associated problems of:

• Swallowing difficulties
• Speech problems
• Visual defects – squint, refractive errors, visual field defects
• Fits
• Constipation
• Vomiting

Management

These children need:

• A multidisciplinary team approach as outlined at the beginning of the chapter
• Continued consultant care
• Continued work with the parents with respite care if necessary
• Therapy to try and achieve maximum use of movements under voluntary control, prevent deformity and encourage mobilization. Therapists may follow a system of care which includes:

> The Bobath Method – the reduction of unwanted and abnormal movements by means of reflex-inhibiting patterns and stretching.
> The Peto system or conductive education. This has been developed in Budapest, Hungary, where one person, a conductor, does all the educational and therapy aspects of the treatment. This has been a controversial method of managing children with cerebral palsy but many British children have gone to Hungary.

The aims of treatment of a child with cerebral palsy include:

• Encouraging correct handling to prevent spasm of hip adductors
• Stretching from a prone board to prevent deformity
• Finding suitable seating

- Using splints and boots where appropriate to prevent deformity
- Selecting a suitable wheelchair where that is indicated
- Liaison with orthopaedic surgeons regarding deformity
- Treating constipation and vomiting

Congenital rubella syndrome

Children with congenital rubella syndrome can suffer from:

- Nerve deafness
- Global developmental delay
- Visual problems, i.e. cataracts and retinal problems

The congenital rubella syndrome has a wide range of variations from mild nerve deafness to the severely multi-handicapped child. Particular attention needs to be made to maximizing the help given to hearing loss so that the child can learn as much as possible. Any visual problem, particularly cataracts, can be dealt with by an ophthalmic surgeon.

These children are often helped by simple sign language such as Makaton.

Down's syndrome

Down's syndrome is one of the commonest recognizable causes of global delay in children. It is due to Trisomy 21 in most cases although there may be rare translocations.

It is important to spend time with the parents at the initial diagnosis and ensure the prognosis is explained. Many Down's syndrome children live a normal life-span and management should encourage children to be as normal as possible.

There are a number of points that need to be considered in the management:

- A programme for the pre-school years needs to be developed including physiotherapy, the Home Advisory Service and speech therapy.
- An echocardiogram should be checked to exclude cardiovascular disease.

- Special weight charts with centiles for Down's syndrome children are available and should be used.
- The parents should have genetic advice.
- Early playgroup or Home Advisory Service is useful.
- The education of children with Down's syndrome is controversial. Many children are now able to be educated in ordinary schools; however, it may be that certain children would be more suitably placed in schools for children with learning difficulties. Many parents feel very strongly that their children should be educated at a normal school and if this is possible they should be encouraged.

Duchenne muscular dystrophy

Duchenne muscular dystrophy is a fairly common disorder in boys with 1 in 4000 male births having the disease. It may present with delayed walking. Two-thirds of the children have significant speech delay. Therefore, the creatine phosphate kinase (CPK) level is always worth checking when the child has speech delay. The diagnosis can usually be made by a grossly elevated serum CPK. Confirmation has traditionally been by muscle biopsy, however, this can now be confirmed by finding deletions in the DNA of the X chromosome using the latest technology.

The problem is of progressive proximal muscle weakness. Most textbooks suggest that the children go into the wheelchair at about the age of 8 years and die in their teenage years. Nowadays many boys do not go into wheelchairs until the age of 10 years or over and many boys managed in a modern way survive into their twenties.

There are a number of different management problems:

- Attention should be paid to the genetics of the condition. The family need referral to an expert in a Regional Genetics Centre. Carrier testing will be needed, the whole family investigated and genetic counselling given. Sisters of affected boys grow up very quickly. Genetic issues should be discussed at each consultation.
- Encourage exercise in the years before a wheelchair is necessary in order to delay the reduction in muscle strength and to prevent obesity. This can be done by encouraging

suitable amounts of walking and by the use of a low geared exercise tricycle (possibly the WRK type).

● Stretching exercises to prevent contractures should be started from an early stage.

● Encourage the adaption of the home before the child goes off his feet. This time is often a very difficult time for the family and dealing with home adaptions may take time and may be difficult to organize.

● Obesity is a major problem with the older boy as calorie requirements are very small in this condition. Attention to the diet is needed from an early stage.

● Scoliosis may develop in the years of the wheelchair. It is cosmetically difficult, makes the patient uncomfortable and reduces respiratory function. Leather or plastic orthotic jackets are helpful, but may not always prevent scoliosis. Operations for scoliosis such as the Luque operation are becoming increasingly established.

● Maintaining ambulation in the boy who has gone off his feet increases morale and may reduce the reduction in muscle power. The upright posture may also help scoliosis. Aids used for this include: long walking callipers, used at the Hammersmith Hospital, and swivel walkers as a low energy form of ambulation.

Learning difficulties

The diagnosis of children with learning difficulties has been dealt with in Chapter 16.

The management of these children in the pre-school years should include:

● Making a diagnosis where possible
● Discussing the diagnosis with parents sensitively
● An ongoing dialogue with the parents
● Genetic advice
● The Home Advisory Service (portage system)
● Physiotherapy and occupational therapy help with mobilization
● Advice on benefits
● Early nursery placement
● Choice of a suitable school

As the child gets older many of the problems are educational rather than medical. Attention needs to be given to:

- Mobilization
- Constipation
- Vomiting
- The control of fits

Osteogenesis imperfecta

There are a number of different types of this condition (see p. 26):

Osteogenesis imperfecta type I

Type I is dominantly inherited usually without deformity. Blue sclerae are seen.

Osteogenesis imperfecta type II

Type II is lethal.

Osteogenesis imperfecta type III

Type III gives severe deformity and needs particular help. The children are growth retarded and may be subject to severe respiratory problems. An electric wheelchair is usually needed. Fractures need to be given support. The use of plastic and inflatable orthoses may be helpful.

Osteogenesis imperfecta type IV

In type IV white sclerae are seen and there is dominant inheritance. Such cases may need help such as in type III.

Neurofibromatosis

This common dominantly inherited condition may present with typical clinical features of the *café au lait* spots. The condition has an importance in childhood because:

- Many children have mild to moderate learning difficulties
- Many children have fits
- Some children have visceral and skin complications of neurofibromatosis: abdominal neurofibromata, optic glioma etc.

Children with neurofibromatosis need on-going paediatric follow-up to recognize problems at an early stage. Since this is also a dominant inherited autosomal condition genetic counselling is indicated.

Prader—Willi syndrome

These children have hypotonia, learning difficulties and hypogonadism. They may become very obese and dietary control is most important. Many of them have a chromosome deletion.

Spina bifida

A reduction of severely deformed children has taken place over the years with antenatal detection and 20% of affected children being selected for closure. The children need an individual planned programme of management with a regular review of aims. Such management includes:

- Dealing with the associated hydrocephalus with valves, either a ventriculo-peritoneal shunt or a ventriculo-atrial shunt. Such a shunt may block or may become infected. A ventriculo-peritoneal shunt requires fewer revisions than an atrial shunt and is now used more often in management.
- Dealing with problems of the bladder and urinary tract. This may include intermittent catheterization, treating infections, urinary diversions, bladder neck surgery and special aids.
- Dealing with constipation which may require regular manual evacuation.
- Attention to genetic issues.
- Attention to mobilization with various orthotic aids such as hip guidance orthoses and orthopaedic surgery.

- Dealing with scoliosis which may require spinal surgery.

Spinal muscular atrophy

There are three types of spinal muscular atrophy.

Severe spinal muscular atrophy or Werdnig Hoffman disease

These children present as severely floppy infants and die in the first 2 years of life from respiratory insufficiency.

Intermediate spinal muscular atrophy

These children again present as floppy infants, but are not as severely affected as in severe spinal muscular atrophy. They tend not to die until their teenage years. Some may have quite long-term survival. They start off being quite severely handicapped and seldom walk. However, the progression of their muscle weakness is only a slow one and their intellect is quite normal. They often appear rather bright children and they are greatly helped by attention to their wheelchair, particularly one of the advanced types of electric wheelchairs. A large clinical problem is a tendency to scoliosis and jacketing needs to be undertaken at an early stage.

Benign spinal muscular atrophy or Kugelberg–Welander syndrome

These children present with muscle weakness which is much slower to progress than intermediate spinal muscular atrophy. They have particular problems with pen work at school and may be helped by an occupational therapist.

The genetics of all these conditions is autosomal recessive and suitable genetic counselling needs to be undertaken.

Tuberose sclerosis

This condition can be very variable and may present with severe global delay and infantile spasms. It may also be a

milder condition with mild learning difficulties or even normal intelligence with skin manifestations of the disease. The
inheritance is a dominant one with a variable penetrance and
a high mutation rate. Linkage studies have been helpful.

Skin manifestations of tuberose sclerosis

The skin manifestations which are most helpful in the first
years of life are depigmented patches or hypomelanic patches
on the skin often in the shape of a leaf, the classical ash leaf
patch. These may be only visible with ultraviolet light. The
skin manifestations of angiofibromata on the face are rarely
obvious till the age of 2 years and may not appear until adult
life. Shagreen patches are large areas of thickened discol-
oured skin of angiofibromatous tissue. Subungual fibromata
may be found.

Other manifestations

As well as skin manifestations there may be fibromatous
lesions in the brain which calcify. The diagnosis can be helped
by looking for intracerebral calcification on CT scan. Half
the patients have learning difficulties. Many children suffer
from seizures of a myoclonic type which may follow infantile
spasms. Regular medical follow-up is indicated for the control
of the convulsions. There may be also rhabdomyomas in the
heart, angiomyolipomas of the kidney, bone cysts and rectal
polyps.

Obtaining equipment for children

Any doctor working with children sometimes needs to obtain
a piece of equipment for a child with special needs. This
may be anything from an outdoor wheelchair to an oxygen
monitor. How should one go about this?

● Always try statutory agencies first. Equipment can often
be obtained from either health or local authority sources.
For instance, always try the local artificial limb and appliance

centre (ALAC) for a wheelchair. Remember that the local social services have responsibility for aids to daily living.

- If equipment cannot be obtained in this way it may be necessary to go to charitable sources. Funds may not be obtained at the first attempt. Try a number of possible sources.

These may be:

- A hospital or health authority trust fund
- The national society for the disease the child is suffering from, e.g. the Spastics Society for a child with cerebral palsy
- Local charities and trusts
- Local organizations such as the Round Table, Lions etc.
- National charities for children such as the Variety Club
- Specific local companies (especially if there is a link with a child or the equipment wanted)

19 Enuresis and soiling

Enuresis

Bed wetting is not a disease, but a variation of normal. The condition affects 10% of 5 year olds and 5% of 10 year olds and, therefore, is very common. A graph of time of becoming dry at night with age has a long tail and enuresis can still be physiological in teenage years. Enuresis is commoner in poorer families and families under stress. There is also very commonly a family history. In many cases there has been day-time wetting for a long period of time.

Excluding organic disease

Although in the vast majority of children there is no neurological or urological cause, it must be remembered that some children with these disorders do present with enuresis. All children over 5 years with enuresis should have:

- Mid-stream urine investigated
- A full history enquiry of such things as constant dribbling etc.
- A full examination, particularly to exclude neurological disease

In some cases, particularly in older children, an examination of their renal tract with an ultrasound scan in the first instance and a micturating cystogram may be indicated. This is not needed in most cases.

Treatment

This condition spontaneously improves with age. All cases must be reassured about the common nature of the problem. There should be an approach of encouraging the child when he or she is dry and without chastisement when the bed is wet. Some important points are:

- Bed wetting should cease being a source of family conversation
- A good washing machine is valuable
- A star chart is valuable in assessing the size of the problem and encouraging dry nights

Other methods available

Drugs

The results of drug treatment in enuresis are disappointing. They may help in the short-term, but not in the long-term.

Tricyclic antidepressants
Tricyclic antidepressants are often advised as the first line of treatment. They have a powerful effect and are dangerous in overdose or when actually taken by younger children. Their use should not be routine, but are sometimes used in particularly acute circumstances.

Desmopressin
Desmopressin may work in the short-term and have less potential side effects than tricyclic antidepressants, but their long-term efficacy is as yet unproven.

Enuresis alarms

With enuresis alarms, when the child passes urine in the bed an alarm sounds and the child gets up and empties the bladder. Although this sounds rather simplistic it often works and should be used as the first line of treatment in most cases.

There are two types of alarms available:

1. A 'pad and bell' which is underneath a sheet
2. A 'body alarm'

Whenever using an enuresis alarm there should be an initial period of assessment with a star chart. If an alarm is going to work it will do so within 5 or 8 weeks. There is little advantage in continuing the therapy for more than 2 months after initial success. Success rates are in the region of just over 50%, but probably their use should be confined to children 7 years old and over.

Dry bed training

This is a training programme which involves being woken hourly and given a high fluid intake for retention controlled training. This is again a technique that works well, particularly under the supervision of a psychologist.

Soiling

There are two main types of soiling that are seen in childhood:

1. Chronic constipation and soiling where the child becomes constipated and there is an overflow with faecal leaking. This is sometimes known as spurious diarrhoea.
2. True encopresis where the child passes whole motions in the pants. This is usually associated with a major behavioural disorder.

Chronic constipation and soiling

This disorder may start with a fissure or with an emotional disorder. There are some children who never become clean and go straight on to this condition. As the constipation becomes more severe a vicious circle starts. The motions become harder and larger and therefore more painful to pass, so the constipation gets worse. The diagnosis is confirmed by:

• A history of constant soiling preceded by constipation
• The faeces being palpable per abdomen
• The faeces being palpable at rectal examination

It should be remembered that very occasionally Hurchsprung's Disease may present in this way.

Aims of treatment

The aims of treatment are:

• To clear the bowel
• To encourage going to the toilet to pass normal motions
• To deal with the emotional problems

The bowel is cleared either by enemas or by strong laxatives such as Picolax. In rare cases the faecal mass may be so large that the only way to deal with the situation is by manual removal under anaesthetic. A hospital admission can be used to do this but is not essential and apart from the manual removal under anaesthetic this can be done as an outpatient.

Laxatives may be needed for some time. A sensible combination to begin with is Lactulose and Senekot, Senekot being gradually reduced first and then the Lactulose. It is essential to encourage the child to continue going to the toilet with continued behavioural help. A star chart with rewards is particularly valuable.

True encopresis

This is a difficult condition and may sometimes be associated with smearing of faeces. It is associated with a major psychological abnormality and needs referral to an expert psychologist or psychiatrist for a detailed analysis of the underlying causes of the problem and a structured programme of treatment.

20 Non-organic problems

Non-organic problems occupy a significant amount of the time of doctors working with children. They are sometimes difficult to diagnose. They also may highlight problems within the family, school environment etc.

Doctors dealing with children with non-organic problems should:

- Make certain of the diagnosis and exclude significant organic differential diagnoses
- Take full social and educational histories

When a diagnosis of a non-organic problem is made emphasize:

- The common nature of the problem
- That it is a real symptom, not a made up one
- That it should improve with simple treatment

Abdominal pain

Abdominal pain is one of the most common non-organic problems in children. This usually occurs before and around puberty. It is rare in children under the age of 5 years. Organic causes for abdominal pain in such children should always be sought and the child should be fully investigated. Girls between the onset of puberty and menarche seem to be particularly liable. The pain is usually central. The further away from the umbilicus the pain is the more likely it is to have an organic cause. The pain is usually short-lived, but may often be fairly frequent.

Differential diagnosis

- Renal disease is usually worth excluding by an ultrasound scan and mid-stream urine (MSU)
- Other investigations need to be done with specific indication, e.g. a barium meal if there is a family history of peptic ulceration, if pain is epigastric
- Constipation by itself is a rare cause of abdominal pain

If possible, care should be taken to make a positive diagnosis of non-organic abdominal pain. The child should be reassured and got back to school as quickly as possible. Doctors should emphasize the willingness to see the child if the pain persists, to admit during an attack as the diagnosis is often much easier to make with abdominal pain, and to discuss the case with other health care professionals and the school if necessary.

Headaches

The boundary between non-organic tension headaches and migraine unfortunately is not a clear one. Headaches due to organic disease can be differentiated usually by history and clinical examination. Skull X-rays and CAT scan are rarely needed, however, they may be useful for reassurance.

Paracetamol is useful. In cases suggestive of migraine Pizotifen is sometimes helpful particularly in cases where there is a positive family history of migraine.

Leg pains

Leg pains are common non-organic pains in younger children. There are stories of a child waking up in the evening with leg pains which are only relieved with time. The old-style paediatrician called these pains growing pains. It had the advantage of sounding natural and reassuring. Investigations are rarely positive. However, if there are prominent calves the creatinine phosphate kinase level (CPK) is sometimes helpful.

Paracetamol is useful. Reassurance is all that is usually needed in these cases.

Vomiting

Recurrent vomiting with no organic cause can be common.

Cyclical vomiting usually has a non-organic basis. If cyclical vomiting is established then children may need to be admitted to hospital during the attack and intravenous fluids given.

Psychological causes for vomiting should be looked for. If there is concern a barium meal and swallow should be done and in some cases a gastroscopy is helpful.

21 Divorce, separation and the child

The divorce or separation of a child's parents has a profound effect on them. It may affect the child's self-image and may alter behaviour and academic performance well into adult life. In many cases also it will alter the financial environment in which the child lives. Living as two households is inevitably more expensive than living as one family and this brings many single-parent families to the poverty level.

As a result of separation or divorce children may present with:

• Behavioural problems. These may particularly be of the temper tantrum type with destructive behaviour as the child subconsciously blames a parent for the break-up of the marriage
• Reduced academic performance
• Non-organic problems such as abdominal pain, headaches etc.
• Child abuse following the introduction of an unsuitable partner into the home

The legal basis of divorce

The grounds for divorce

The law (the *Matrimonial Causes Act* 1973) looks at whether there has been an irretrievable breakdown in a marriage or not. It places a duty on legal advisors to attempt reconciliation between the parties if possible. Grounds for the irretrievable breakdown include:

- Adultery which the petitioner finds intolerable
- Unreasonable behaviour
- The husband and wife have lived apart for 2 years (with consent) or 5 years (without consent)

In practice often the parties have agreed that a divorce is inevitable and agree the grounds.

Cases are heard at the county court. They are heard before judges and if children are involved the court has to be satisfied that the arrangements for them are satisfactory. The court may order the probation service, the local authority or any other person to make a welfare report on the children.

Financial arrangements are also dealt with by the court. Although theoretically independent of the arrangements for the children, which parent they live with has a major effect on the ultimate settlement.

If the grounds are proved and the court has dealt with the arrangements for the children and finance, it will grant a *decree nisi*. This will convert to a *decree absolute* on application from one of the parties from 6 weeks after the *decree nisi*.

Legal arrangements for the children

The *Children Act* 1989 makes major changes in the private law regarding children. It introduces a concept of parental responsibility which replaces parental rights and duties. Parental responsibility is defined as 'all the rights, duties, powers, responsibilities and authority that a parent has in relation to a child and his property'. Although this language perhaps does not make it clear, it is intended that parental responsibility is largely concerned with matters of upbringing such as education, medical treatment and religion. In all cases the interests of the child come first.

Under the *Children Act* 1989 the court can decide the following private law orders which should be flexible to deal with the requirements of individual children:

- The person with whom a child should live (residence orders)
- Any form of contact he or she should have with other people (contact orders)
- Any other particular matter concerning the child (specific issue orders)
- Anything that should be prohibited from being done in relation to the child (prohibited steps order)

Difference between parental responsibility and residence

Many parents and professionals are confused by these different concepts in law. There are two major decisions that need to be made for a child:

- Where he or she lives
- Who has responsibility for the important decisions about that child's welfare (i.e. education, religion, medical treatment)

The decision about where a child lives is made by the court by granting a residence order. In the law before the *Children Act* 1989 this was called care and control. In most cases this is given to the mother although there is no reason why a father should not be given residence in most cases.

The decision about who has 'parental responsibility' for the child is also confirmed by the court. A parent can live away from the child but still have parental responsibility. Before the *Children Act* 1989 the similar concept was called 'custody'. It was possible to have joint custody of a child and to have custody but not care and control.

Before the *Children Act* 1989 the court decided what 'access' arrangements should be made for the parent who did not have care and control. With the new law the court makes contact orders. The court also has discretion to grant any other of the Section 8 orders if it feels it is in the interest of the child.

The doctor's role

Clearly it would be important to prevent marriage break-up if possible because of the unhappiness it causes to both the parents and to the children. This may not always be possible. Doctors are often asked for their advice regarding the arrangements for the children after divorce and in particular for reports on the effect of a particular illness on those arrangements. Many doctors get confused regarding the legal basis of divorce and confused regarding advice they should give regarding parental responsibility and contact orders.

The role of the children's doctor in divorce may be:

- Counselling to prevent marriage breakdown
- Advising regarding the arrangements for the children
- Conciliation between parties after divorce

The doctor's role before marriage break-up

A child may present with behavioural problems or non-organic symptoms and on investigation the cause is found to be the impending break-up of the parents' marriage. In these cases it may be appropriate to counsel the parents and to help them restore their previous relationship.

Marriage counselling is a skilled matter and most doctors may find themselves out of their depth in helping such parents. Help can be obtained from:

- RELATE: The Marriage Guidance Council (see local telephone directory)
- A local psychologist or psychiatrist who has a particular interest in such counselling

It may be there are specific problems within the family, for instance, financial or psychosexual problems that need specific help.

The doctor's role during the divorce

The doctor may be asked for a report regarding the arrangements for the children by the court (usually via the probation service). This is usually regarding specific health matters. These reports should state:

- The condition from which the child suffers
- The prognosis

• How it would be affected by residential alternatives for the child

If possible the report should be concise and factual and not take sides.

Doctors may also be asked advice by parents regarding these residential and contact arrangements. There are clear principles that apply:

• Contact should be maintained with both parents if at all possible
• Both parents should be involved in major decisions about the child, i.e. they both should have parental responsibility
• There should be regular contact with the parent the child does not live with, even if that contact is infrequent
• The contact arrangements should include overnight stays if possible
• Disputes regarding finance or the cause of the marriage breakdown should not affect the contact arrangements

In practice it may be very difficult for fathers to remain in contact with their children. They may not have a suitable place to take the child for contact. There may also be financial or geographical reasons why contact is difficult. All these problems may become insurmountable in poor families and many fathers unfortunately lose contact with their children.

The doctor's role after the divorce

Children may present with similar behavioural problems after the divorce as before it. These may be compounded by problems with the introduction of a step-parent into the home. Maintaining an on-going relationship with the parent who lives away from the home continues to be important.

Parents may be helped in some areas by the Conciliation Service. The aim of this service is not to restore the parents' previous relationship but to get them to agree mutually satisfactory contact and residential arrangements which will benefit the children with the help of a third party.

Appendix

Organizations helping children and supporting families with special needs

• Action Research for the Crippled Child, Vincent House, North Parade, Horsham, West Sussex RH12 2DA. Telephone 0403-64101

• Arthritis and Rheumatism Council for Research, 41 Eagle Street, London WC1 4AR. Telephone 071-405 8572

• Association for all Speech Impaired Children, 347 Central Market, Smithfield, London EC1 9NH. Telephone 071-236 6478

• Association for Spina Bifida and Hydrocephalus, 22 Upper Woburn Place, London WC1 0EP. Telephone 071-388 1382

• Barnardo's, Tanner's Lane, Barkingside, Ilford, Essex IG6 1QG. Telephone 081-550 8822

• British Paediatric Association, 5 St Andrews Place, London NW1 4LB. Telephone 071-486 6151

• British Bone Society, 112 City Road, Dundee DD2 2PW. Telephone 0382-67603

• British Association for Community Child Health (formerly Community Paediatric Group) Community Health Department, Newbridge Hill, Bath BA1 3QE

• Disabled Living Foundation, 380–384 Harrow Road, London W9 2HU. Telephone 071-289 6111

• Down's Syndrome Association, 12–13 Clapham Common, Southside, London SW4 7AA. Telephone 071-720 0008

• Haemophilia Society, 123 Westminster Bridge Road, London SE1 7HR. Telephone 071-928 2020

• Muscular Dystrophy Group for Great Britain and Northern Ireland, Nattrass House, 35 Macauley Road, London SW4 0QP. Telephone 071-720 8055

• National Children's Bureau, 8 Wakely Street, London EC1V 7QE. Telephone 071-278 9441

• National Deaf Children's Society, 45 Hereford Road, London W2 5AH. Telephone 071-229 9272/4

• National Meningitis Trust, Fern House, Bath Road, Stroud, Glos GL5 3TJ. Telephone 0453-751738

• Pre-School Playgroups Association, 61–63 King's Cross Road, London WC1X 9LL. Telephone 071-833 8991

• Research Trust for Metabolic Diseases in Children, 53 Beam Street, Nantwich, Cheshire CW5 5NF. Telephone 0270-629782

• Royal National Institute for the Blind, 224 Great Portland Street, London W1N 6AA. Telephone 071-388 1266

• Royal National Institute for the Deaf, 105 Gower Street, London WC1 6AH. Telephone 071-387 8033

• Soft UK, Support Organisation for Trisomy 13/18
Trisomy 13, Jenny Robbins, Tudor Lodge, Redwood, Ross-on-Wye, Herefordshire HR9 5UD. Telephone 0989-67480

Trisomy 18, Christine Rose, 48 Froggats Ride, Walmley, Sutton Coldfield, West Midlands B76 8TQ. Telephone 021-351 3122

• Spastics Society, 12 Park Crescent, London W1N 4EQ. Telephone 071-636 5020

• SANDS, Stillbirth and Neonatal Death Society, 28 Portland Place, London W1N 4DE. Telephone 071-436 5861

• Twins and Multiple Births Association, 20 Redcar Close, Lillington, Leamington Spa CV32 7SU. Telephone 0926-22688

Bibliography

Progress in Child Health, Volume 1 (1984) and Volumes 2 and 3 (1985), edited by J.A. McFarlane. Many useful articles on a variety of aspects of community child health.

British Asians: Health in the Community, Patience Karseras and Eirwen Hopkins, John Wiley and Sons, Chichester, 1987. Good guide to the social background and health of British Asians.

An Introduction to the Children Act 1989, HMSO, London. The Act itself is difficult to understand. This makes it clearer.

Children: The New Law, Andrew Bainham, Family Law, 1990. A readable guide to the legal aspects of the Children Act 1989.

ABC of Child Abuse, edited by Roy Meadow, British Medical Journal, 1989. A readable guide to child abuse with good illustrations.

Diagnosis of Child Sexual Abuse: Guidance for Doctors, HMSO, 1988, and *Physical Signs of Sexual Abuse in Children*, 1991, Royal College of Physicians. Both clear guides to practice in this difficult subject.

154

Immunisation against Infectious Disease, 1990, Dept of Health, the Welsh Office, Scottish Home and Health Department. HMSO. An important guide to good immunization practice. Revised yearly.

Adopting a Child, Prue Chennells and Chris Hammond, 1990, British Agencies for Fostering and Adoption. Advice for couples wishing to adopt. Much useful information for the professional.

Sudden Death in Infancy, Bernard Knight, Faber and Faber, London, 1983. Many facts about the Sudden Infant Death Syndrome.

Health for All Children, edited by David Hall, Oxford Medical Publications. The report of the working party on child surveillance.

Child Health Surveillance in Primary Care. A Critical Review, HMSO. John Butler.

The Child with a Handicap, David Hall, Blackwell Medical Publications, 1984. A splendid book with much useful advice on the assessment, treatment and diagnosis of handicap in children.

Neurologically Handicapped Children: Treatment and Management, Neil Gordon and Ian McKinley, Blackwell, 1986. A useful guide to the management of neurological conditions.

Language, Development and Disorders, edited by William Yule and Michael Rutter, Clinics in Developmental Medicine, 1987. A very detailed guide to a complex subject.

Child and Adolescent Psychiatry. Modern Approaches, edited by Michael Rutter and Lionel Hersov, Blackwell. A detailed and useful textbook.

Smith's Patterns of Human Malformation, fourth edition, Kenneth Lyon Jones, W.B. Saunders, 1988. An invaluable guide to patterns of malformation.

Matrimonial Proceedings, Richard Davies and Marilyn Mornington, Longman, 1988. A good account of divorce law.

Index

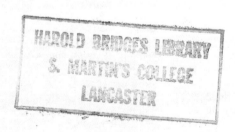